PRACTICAL
I. V. Therapy
SECOND EDITION

PRACTICAL

I. V. Therapy

SECOND EDITION

JULIE STEELE, RN
I.V. Therapy Education Coordinator
Tallahassee, Florida

Springhouse Corporation
Springhouse, Pennsylvania

STAFF

Senior Publisher
Minnie B. Rose, RN, BSN, MEd

Art Director
John Hubbard

Clinical Editors
Patricia Kardish Fischer, RN, BSN;
Maryann Foley, RN, BSN

Editors
Diane Labus, David Moreau

Copy Editor
Diane M. Armento

Designers
Stephanie Peters (senior associate art
director), Lorraine Lostracco,
Susan Hopkins Rodzewich

Typography
Diane Paluba (manager), Elizabeth Bergman,
Joyce Rossi Biletz, Phyllis Marron, Valerie L.
Rosenberger

Manufacturing
Deborah Meiris (director), T.A. Landis,
Andreas Hess

Editorial Assistants
Jeanne Napier, Louise Quinn, Betsy K.
Snyder

The clinical procedures described and recommended in this publication are based on currently accepted clinical theory and practice and on consultation with medical and nursing authorities. Nevertheless, they cannot be considered absolute and universal recommendations. For individual application, all recommendations must be considered in light of the patient's clinical condition and, before administration of new or infrequently used drugs, in light of the latest package-insert information. The author and the publisher disclaim responsibility for any adverse effects resulting directly or indirectly from the suggested procedures, from any undetected errors, or from the reader's misunderstanding of the text.

Printed in the United States of America.

PIVT2E-011195

℞ A member of the Reed Elsevier plc group

Library of Congress Cataloging-in-Publication Data
Steele, Julie.
  Practical I.V. therapy/Julie Steele. — 2nd ed.
     p.   cm.
  Includes bibliographical references and index.
  1. Intravenous therapy—Handbooks, manuals,
etc. 2. Nursing—Handbooks, manuals, etc.   I. Title.
  [DNLM: 1. Infusions, Intravenous—nursing.
WY150 S814p 1996]
RM170.S74 1996
615'.6—dc20
DNLM/DLC   95-37817
ISBN 0-87434-784-X (alk. paper)   CIP

DEDICATION

To nurses dealing with I.V. therapy in these changing times. Remember, keep it practical, but more so keep it, and you, safe.

To Kevin Soike, RN, BSN, for all his love and inspiration both spiritually and professionally.

To my children, Robert and Andrea, for challenging me.

Special thanks to Julie Brujin, RN; Telia Cunningham, RPh; Guy Ellis, RPh; and Joan Alford, RN, for their help in revising the information in this edition.

DEDICATION

CONTENTS

PREFACE

Practical I.V. Therapy, Second Edition is a practical, hands-on resource containing current recommendations and guidelines in accordance with the Centers for Disease Control and the Intravenous Nurses Society for many aspects of I.V. therapy. Written by an I.V. nurse with many years of practical experience, this book offers a no-nonsense approach to an often-misunderstood area of nursing.

Commonly thought of as the mere insertion of I.V. needles, I.V. therapy involves much more, including infection control, maintaining fluid and electrolyte balance, and assessing for potential complications. *Practical I.V. Therapy, Second Edition* covers these areas and offers helpful hints about starting, maintaining, and discontinuing I.V. lines. All of the chapters have been updated using the most current information about solutions, equipment, safety measures, and guidelines.

The appendices present nursing care plans, a discussion of continuous quality improvement in I.V. therapy, problem solving for real-life situations with explanatory answers, and standardization of I.V. care.

Although this book is not designed to answer all questions about I.V. therapy, it provides a practical, useful means to better I.V. skills, thereby improving the quality of patient care.

1

INTRODUCTION TO I.V. THERAPY

One of your most important responsibilities as a nurse will be to administer fluids, medications, and blood products to patients in various clinical settings. For example, a postoperative patient who has undergone major abdominal surgery may require an infusion to replace fluids and electrolytes. A child with severe asthma or a diabetic patient with an infected ulcer may need intravenous (I.V.) medications. A victim of a multiple-vehicle accident may die without a blood transfusion. And a cancer patient may need repeated courses of chemotherapy to lessen the effects of the disease.

I.V. therapy is the introduction of therapeutic liquid agents directly into the venous circulation. It enables health care providers to ensure adequate hydration, to maintain fluid and electrolyte homeostasis, and to administer medications, radiographic dyes, chemotherapeutic agents, nutritional supplements, and blood and blood products necessary for sustaining life or correcting complications.

Administered properly, I.V. therapy is a lifeline. However, improper technique can lead to inflamed veins, swollen limbs, tissue sloughing, and impaired feeling or circulation. Problems can occur whenever the skin is penetrated, so asepsis is crucial to prevent bacterial infiltration. The introduction of bacteria into the bloodstream is extremely serious; for a patient who is already sick or immunosuppressed, it can be fatal.

As a nurse, you will have to make decisions about which I.V. equipment to use based on your patient's condition and the type of solution to be administered. You will need to know how to set up this equipment and to select an appropriate venipuncture site. You will be responsible for starting and discontinuing I.V. lines in patients of all ages and for ensuring their comfort and safety throughout therapy. And you will need to monitor carefully for signs and symptoms of complications.

INFECTION CONTROL
Controlling infection is of paramount importance in I.V. therapy. Because I.V. fluids are an invasion of the body's closed internal system, precautions are necessary to ensure that this infiltration is advantageous to the patient. Infection-control measures help prevent bacteria from entering the circulation and spreading disease during I.V. therapy. Many hospitals are staffed with infection-control nurses, who monitor the spread of disease and educate other staff members about effective infection-control measures. However, because infection-control nurses are not found in all facilities, *all* nurses are responsible for using safe practices to prevent the spread of disease.

Hand washing, one of the most effective ways to prevent the transmission of disease-causing bacteria, is perhaps the most valuable tool in infection control. The mere use of soap and water combined with friction is so basic, yet so very important. However, this simple technique is often done ineffectively and, in some cases, neglected entirely.

The Occupational Safety and Health Administration (OSHA), a major force in the fight for tight infection-control measures and safety in the workplace, has established strict guidelines that address the transmission of blood-borne and airborne pathogens among health care professionals and their patients. Such guidelines are necessary and can be lifesaving, especially in light of the risks posed by the hepatitis B virus and human immunodeficiency virus (HIV), the causative agent of acquired immunodeficiency syndrome (AIDS).

Until AIDS became such a major health issue, health care professionals focused mainly on protecting their patients from communicating the disease. However, the growing threat of the AIDS epidemic has forced the health care community to take a more introspective look at its own safety. In the late 1980s, the Centers for Disease Control (CDC) published its first set of universal blood and body fluid precautions regarding the transmission of HIV and other transmittable diseases. In 1991, OSHA issued a standard on blood-borne pathogens, mandating the use of Universal Precautions in all health care settings.

Universal Precautions eliminated much of the guesswork about how to handle patients with potentially communicable diseases. Previously, many patients were placed in disease-specific isolation until a positive diagnosis could be made. However, this type of isolation was effective only when laboratory tests positively confirmed the suspected diagnosis; in some cases, patients were inadvertently placed in the wrong type of isolation, further increasing the risk of transmitting disease to health care workers and other patients in the same isolation units.

Universal Precautions offers health care professionals a new means of protection against infection and a new approach to fighting the spread of disease:
- Treat *all* body fluids and secretions as if they are infectious by avoiding direct contact with them.
- Use protective equipment, such as gloves, when providing patient care.
- Wash hands thoroughly after removing protective equipment.

Although wearing gloves is an effective way to guard against infection, I.V. nurses must take care to select the most appropriate and effective type of gloves. Allergies to latex or the powder in gloves are common, and any break in the skin is an excellent breeding ground for bacterial growth. If you note itchy rash, burning skin, or swelling, consult your supervisor immediately because the facility is responsible for providing you with the proper protective gear.

Remember, gloves are *not* meant to replace hand washing, but they do offer another means of preventing contamination when providing I.V. therapy. Thorough hand cleansing before and after performing a procedure is the primary infection-prevention step. However, you may find it necessary to wash again during the procedure to prevent contamination.

I.V. therapy has been associated with the development of nosocomial bacteremia. These hospital-associated infections prolong hospital stays by several days and increase overall medical costs. After years of research in all medical fields, including I.V. therapy, the CDC has established procedural guidelines to promote continuity of care and to prevent and control such infections. Some hospitals staff I.V. teams with specially trained nurses to enforce these policies and procedures and to ensure quality I.V. care. However, because I.V. teams are not available in some facilities, all nurses must know and follow CDC guidelines when providing I.V. therapy (see *Infection Control in I.V. Therapy,* pages 4 and 5, for CDC recommendations for treatment and prevention of major infections.)

The incidence of nosocomial bacteremia caused by extrinsically contaminated I.V. fluid (fluid contaminated in hospital settings) is unknown, but it appears to be quite low — at least 10 times lower than the incidence of endemic cannula-related septicemia (contamination that occurs during the manufacturing process). Distinguishing intrinsic contamination from extrinsic contamination can be difficult; however, regardless of the cause of the contamination, the criteria for determining whether contamination has occurred remain the same:

● recovery of the same infection-causing species from cultures of infusate and from blood cultures obtained by separate venipuncture, with a negative semiquantitative culture of the cannula
● lack of another identifiable source of septicemia
● clinical manifestations consistent with bloodstream infection.

Carrying out infection-control policies protects everyone and begins with practicing proper hand-washing techniques. This cannot be overstated, because most device-related cases of septicemia are caused by the patient's own skin flora or by microorganisms transmitted from the hands of the person inserting the device.

Future success in reducing the number of reported nosocomial infections will depend greatly on the implementation of infection-control techniques and the commitment of a team approach to all aspects of I.V. care. Nurses must take the initiative and attend in-service education classes regularly to stay current in this area of nursing. Also, consulting the hospital's infection-control nurse about potential problems and concerns ensures the use of effective, up-to-date infection-control practices.

VENOUS ACCESS DEVICES

The equipment used to access veins depends on where the device is to be inserted and its intended purpose. Therefore, it is important to know what you are using and what potential risks may be involved.

Two types of venous access devices are available: peripheral devices (which access the veins in the head, arms, hands, and feet) and central devices (which access the central venous system more directly, such as through the jugular, subclavian, or femoral vein). An infection in either location (peripheral or central) can lead to sepsis; however, infection caused by peripheral access site is easier to identify and eliminate to prevent sepsis.

Every type of cannula has the potential to cause a bacteremic infection. Plastic cannulas may present a greater hazard than steel ones,

INFECTION CONTROL IN I.V. THERAPY

The chart below provides typical causes and signs and symptoms of the two major categories of infection associated with I.V. therapy, along with Centers for Disease Control recommendations for treatment and prevention.

Type of contamination	Causes	Signs and symptoms
Microbial contamination of infusate (usually gramnegative bacilli)	• Contamination during manufacturing (intrinsic) • Contamination during hospital preparation (extrinsic)	• Signs and symptoms of sepsis — fever, chills, headache, general malaise, and sweats — begin shortly after infusion is started. • Antibiotics fail to resolve infection as long as infusion continues. • Rapid improvement occurs with discontinuation of I.V. fluid. • Same organism is isolated from infusate and patient's blood. • No obvious local infection occurs.
I.V.-related infections	• Absence of or improper hand-washing technique • Inadequate site preparation • Poor cannula insertion technique • Poor site care and lack of antibiotic or antiseptic ointment • Cracks and disconnections in equipment open the system to infection • Poor technique in accessing ports for piggyback medications	• Redness is noted. • Pain or tenderness occurs. • Fever may be present. • Purulent drainage from I.V. site exists.

and central lines may be more hazardous than peripheral lines. Bacteremic infections can be greatly reduced by knowing the possible causes and methods to prevent infection and by implementing routine, meticulous, aseptic I.V. care.

Peripheral lines

Peripheral access can be accomplished using steel needles or plastic cannulas. The lowest incidence of cannula-related infection has been reported with steel needles, although steel needles are not as widely used as plastic cannulas. The potential for infiltration and the frequency

Treatment	Prevention
● If fluid contamination is suspected, the I.V. infusion should be discontinued, the fluid cultured, and the implicated bottle saved. ● Send bottle to laboratory for analysis. ● Continual assessment of patient's vital signs is necessary.	● Control solution exposure to hospital pathogens. ● Use laminar flow hoods to decrease airborne contaminants. ● Have trained personnel handle solutions and carry out aseptic technique. ● Assure quality control process in manufacturing. ● Observe solutions for particulate matter, discoloration, check for expired solutions, and look for cracks in bottles before use.
● Culture I.V. site for purulent drainage, purulent cellulitis, and fever of unknown origin. ● Remove cannula when sepsis is suspected; save and culture. ● Entire I.V. system should be changed upon detection of purulent drainage. ● Cannula should be changed if phlebitis occurs without other signs of infection. ● Retain for 24 hours any I.V. line that is discontinued because of a red, painful, or irritated vein. Milk site for drainage that is not visible; obtain drainage specimen for culture and document, if noted.	● Maintain good hand-washing practices and wear gloves. ● Maintain aseptic technique. ● Develop good insertion technique. ● Secure and protect the cannula and I.V. site. ● Perform regular maintenance: observe site every time you enter patient's room; palpate site for pain and venous texture; rotate I.V. site (every 48 to 72 hours); and maintain routine site care. ● Change I.V. system every 48 hours to prevent contamination from manipulation, as occurs with injecting medications and flushing lines. ● Avoid unnecessary system interruption or penetration. ● Limit added equipment. Each junction provides an opening for bacteria to enter. ● Use strict aseptic technique when medications are given by piggyback or I.V. push.

for restarting the I.V. line are much higher with steel needles.

Plastic cannulas probably place the patient at higher risk for infection than steel needles for routine I.V. therapy simply because they are more likely to remain in one location for prolonged periods. However, they usually are safer for many other aspects of I.V. therapy, such as insertion and maintenance. The newer materials also tend to be more vein-friendly.

Note: Device-related septicemia does not occur in patients with steel or plastic cannulas when the device is inserted under aseptic conditions and removed within 72 hours. After 72 hours, the potential for infection increases dramatically.

Central lines

Central venous access can be accomplished using single- or multiple-lumen subclavian catheters, Swan-Ganz catheters, jugular catheters, or femoral catheters. Regardless of the catheter's intended purpose, it is important to remember that the subclavian, femoral, and jugular veins are very close to the heart's direct circulation. In many cases, the tip of the catheter lies in the superior vena cava or near the entrance to the right atrium. Consequently, bacteria in these catheters can cause sepsis, which poses an immediate threat to the patient.

Consistent, meticulous cannula care lessens the need to replace subclavian or internal jugular cannulas at prespecified intervals. However, when a cannula must be inserted through a burn wound, it should be replaced every third day.

Another type of central access device is the peripherally inserted central cather (PICC). It consists of a highly flexible silastic cannula that is inserted (usually by an RN) into an antecubital vein and a catheter that is fed through the upper one-third of the superior vena cava. The tip of the catheter lies in the superior vena cava or near the entrance to the right atrium. This catheter, which is placed under sterile technique, is less expensive than a surgically implanted central catheter line. The key to preventing infection with this device is fastidious site care and secure catheter connection.

Surgically implanted lines, infusion ports, and infusion pumps

Surgically implanted lines are usually central in location and include the Hickman and Groshong catheters. These devices are inserted under the skin in the chest and tunneled to a central site. A Dacron cuff positioned under the skin on the subcutaneous portion of a silastic cannula seems to add an extra element of protection against extrinsic infection, serving as a barrier that inhibits bacteria from entering the bloodstream from the exit site. Because bacteria would have to migrate past the Dacron cuff and up the tunneled catheter to reach the entrance of the vessel, the cuff makes sepsis from the exit site less likely (assuming the exit site is well maintained).

Surgically implanted infusion ports are central lines consisting of a silastic catheter attached to a port that is placed under the skin. The port must be accessed from outside the body to infuse I.V. solution or remove blood. The risk of infection is in the surgical procedure itself and in the technique used to access the port. Sterile technique is essential.

Surgically implanted infusion pumps consist of a silastic catheter attached to a pump device that is surgically implanted under the skin. These are used to administer chemotherapeutic agents or pain medications continuously in very small quantities. The infection risk is much like that of implanted ports: the pump must be surgically implanted and accessed from outside the body, which increases the risk of infection. Therefore, sterile technique is essential.

FLUIDS AND ELECTROLYTES
A review of normal fluid and electrolyte balance is necessary to understand and implement I.V. therapy. This, along with a working knowledge of the various I.V. fluids available for maintaining normal fluid and electrolyte balance, helps ensure optimum patient care.

All body fluids, including those in intracellular and extracellular compartments, contain various amounts of water and solute, such as anions and cations (electrolytes). These fluids account for approximately 67% of the total body weight in an adult (approximately 70 kg) and roughly 75% of the body weight in an infant. Adipose tissue contains less water than any other type of tissue in the body, so obese persons and females, who usually have a greater portion of adipose tissue, have a lower percentage of body fluids per total body weight.

The total fluid intake requirement of a normal, healthy adult is estimated at 2,300 ml/day. A large portion typically is ingested in the form of pure water, beverages, or food. About 150 to 250 ml of water is synthesized daily in the body through metabolic processes. To maintain homeostasis, or normal balance, the body eliminates the same amount of fluid daily through urine (about 1,400 ml), feces (about 100 ml), perspiration (about 100 ml), and insensible perspiration via the respiratory tract (about 350 ml) and skin (about 350 ml).

Body water, one component of body fluid, serves many important functions. It acts as a structural component and cushion for cells, as a solvent in digestion and excretion, as a lubricant, as a body temperature regulator, and as a medium for all other body fluids and metabolism. Water is also important as a transporter of other substances. Problems occur when the normal balance of the proportions of water and solutes is altered.

All body fluids are contained in two different compartments: the intracellular space and the extracellular space. The intracellular fluid (ICF) compartment includes all of the fluid found within the cells of the body. The extracellular fluid (ECF) compartment includes all of the fluid found outside the cells, including intravascular fluid (blood plasma) and interstitial fluid (fluid found between the cells). Each compartment contains water and electrolytes in specific concentrations. For example, more sodium is contained in ECF than in ICF, whereas more potassium is found in ICF than in ECF. (For a breakdown of the differences related to each compartment, see *Intracellular-Extracellular Concentrations and Serum Laboratory Values,* page 8.)

INTRACELLULAR-EXTRACELLULAR CONCENTRATIONS AND SERUM LABORATORY VALUES

Agents	Normal concentrations		Normal serum laboratory values
	Intracellular	Extracellular	
Na^+	10 mEq/liter*	142 mEq/liter	135 to 145 mEq/liter
K^+	140 mEq/liter	4 mEq/liter	3.5 to 5.2 mEq/liter
Ca^{++}	<1 mEq/liter	5 mEq/liter	8.5 to 10.5 mg/dl
Mg^{++}	58 mEq/liter	3 mEq/liter	1.5 to 3.5 mEq/liter
Cl^-	4 mEq/liter	103 mEq/liter	100 to 106 mEq/liter
HCO_3^-	10 mEq/liter	28 mEq/liter	24 to 31 mEq/liter
pH	7.0	7.4	7.35 to 7.45
Osmolality			280 to 294 mOsm/kg

*mEq is the measure of the chemical-combining power of an ion with hydrogen.

Serum osmolarity refers to the number of osmols, the standard unit of osmotic pressure (the number of water molecules in relation to the number of particles in solution), per liter of solution; it is measured in mOsm/liter of solution. Serum osmolality refers to the number of osmoles per kilogram of solvent; it is measured in mOsm/kg water. Although the terms are slightly different, they often are used interchangeably.

A change in the number of particles alters the chemical-combining ability of the water. The composition of body fluids in the intracellular and extracellular compartments changes as movement across a semipermeable membrane occurs. This membrane selectively allows water and particles to exchange between compartments; any change in one compartment produces a change in the other. Transport mechanisms, such as diffusion and osmosis, affect the movement of solutes (particles) and water through these compartments.

Special functions of major electrolytes

Six major electrolytes—sodium, potassium, calcium, chloride, phosphorus, and magnesium—play important roles in maintaining chemical balance in the body (see *Major Electrolytes,* pages 10 and 11).

- *Sodium* (Na^+) directly affects the balance of water in intracellular and extracellular spaces and controls the distribution of water throughout the body. Fluid volume is altered whenever sodium concentration changes. An important relationship among sodium, chloride, and bicarbonate electrolytes exists; any disturbance in the balance of one affects the other two. Sodium is essential for neuromuscular impulse transmission and contraction. It regulates acid-base balance by combining with chloride and bicarbonate and facilitates numerous chemical reactions.
- *Potassium* (K^+) is essential to neuromuscular impulse transmission and muscle contraction. It controls intracellular osmotic pressure, assists with transporting glucose into the cell, and helps maintain acid-base balance by exchanging with hydrogen ions across the cell membrane.
- *Calcium* (Ca^{++}) alters the cell membrane's permeability and is responsible for proper conduction of electrical impulses and muscle contractility of cardiac, skeletal, and smooth muscles. Necessary for proper blood clotting, calcium also provides a foundation for bones and teeth and helps regulate metabolic enzyme activity.
- *Chloride* (Cl^-) helps regulate acid-base balance by acting as a chemical buffer and by competing with bicarbonate ions for sodium. It influences fluid volume by maintaining extracellular osmotic pressure (keeping fluid outside cells).
- *Phosphate* (P^{--}) is a critical component of general cellular metabolism and energy exchanges (for example, the adenosine triphosphate [ATP] and enzyme systems). It is a building block of the cell membrane (such as in phospholipids) and a structural component of bone. It also plays a major role in the renal excretion of hydrogen ions to maintain acid-base balance.
- *Magnesium* (Mg^{++}) plays a major role in cellular metabolism by facilitating the release of energy from ATP when it is converted to adenosine diphosphate (ADP). It also regulates cellular potassium exchange through the sodium-potassium pump and influences Ca^+ levels via parathyroid hormone secretion (decreases Mg^{++} and Ca^+). It acts as a sedative on neuromuscular transmission and is required for proper enzyme activity in glucose metabolism and protein synthesis.

Note: An increase or decrease in serum calcium level is associated with the opposite change in serum phosphate level.

MAJOR ELECTROLYTES

Electrolytes dissociate in solution into electrically charged particles called ions that have either a negative charge (anions) or a positive charge (cations). Within each body compartment, the number of cations must equal the number of anions to achieve a chemical balance. A loss or gain of electrolytes and an increase or decrease in body fluid can affect this delicate chemical balance.

Six major electrolytes play important roles in maintaining chemical balance. Electrolyte concentrations are expressed in milliequivalents (mEq) and millimoles (mmol).

Electrolyte	Principal functions	Signs and symptoms of imbalance
Sodium (Na⁺) • Major cation in extracellular fluid (ECF) • Normal serum level: 135 to 145 mEq/liter (135 to 145 mmol/liter)	• Maintains appropriate ECF osmolarity • Influences water distribution (with chloride) • Affects concentration, excretion, and absorption of potassium and chloride • Helps regulate acid-base balance • Aids nerve- and muscle-fiber impulse transmission	*Hyponatremia:* muscle weakness, decreased skin turgor, headache, tremor, and seizures *Hypernatremia:* thirst, fever, flushed skin, oliguria, and dry, sticky membranes
Potassium (K⁺) • Major cation in intracellular fluid (ICF) • Normal serum level: 3.5 to 5.2 mEq/liter (3.5 to 5.2 mmol/liter)	• Maintains cell electroneutrality • Maintains cell osmolarity • Assists in conduction of nerve impulses • Directly affects cardiac muscle contraction • Plays major role in acid-base balance	*Hypokalemia:* decreased GI, skeletal muscle, and cardiac muscle function; decreased reflexes; rapid, weak, irregular pulse; muscle weakness or irritability; decreased blood pressure; nausea and vomiting; and paralytic ileus *Hyperkalemia:* muscle weakness, nausea, diarrhea, oliguria
Calcium (Ca⁺⁺) • Major cation in teeth and bones • Normal serum level: 8.5 to 10.5 mg/dl	• Enhances bone strength and durability • Helps maintain cell-membrane structure, function, and permeability • Affects activation, excitation, and contraction of cardiac and skeletal muscles • Participates in neurotransmitter release at synapses • Helps activate specific steps in blood coagulation • Activates serum complement in immune system function	*Hypocalcemia:* muscle tremor, muscle cramps, tetany, tonic-clonic seizures, paresthesia, bleeding, arrhythmias, and hypotension *Hypercalcemia:* lethargy, headache, muscle flaccidity, nausea, vomiting, anorexia, constipation, polydipsia, hypertension, and polyuria

MAJOR ELECTROLYTES *(continued)*		
Electrolyte	**Principal functions**	**Signs and symptoms of imbalance**
Chloride (Cl⁻) $^{}$ • Major anion in ECF • Normal serum level: 100 to 106 mEq/liter (100 to 106 mmol/liter)	• Maintains serum osmolarity (along with Na⁺) • Combines with major cations to create important compounds, such as sodium chloride (NaCl), hydrogen chloride (HCl), potassium chloride (KCl), and calcium chloride (CaCl₂)	*Hypochloremia:* increased muscle excitability, tetany, and decreased respirations *Hyperchloremia:* stupor, rapid deep breathing, and muscle weakness
Phosphate (P⁻⁻) • Major anion in ICF • Normal serum level: 2.5 to 5.0 mEq/dl (0.80 to 1.60 mmol/liter)	• Helps maintain bones and teeth • Helps maintain cell integrity • Plays major role in acid-base balance (as a urinary buffer) • Promotes energy transfer to cells • Plays essential role in muscle, red blood cell, and neurologic functions	*Hypophosphatemia:* paresthesia (circumoral and peripheral), lethargy, and speech defects (such as stuttering or stammering) *Hyperphosphatemia:* renal failure; vague neuroexcitability ranging from tetany to seizures; arrhythmias and muscle twitching with sudden rise in phosphate level
Magnesium (Mg⁺⁺) • Major cation in ICF (closely related to Ca⁺⁺ and P⁻⁻) • Normal serum level: 1.3 to 3.5 mEq/liter with 33% bound to protein and remainder as free cations	• Activates intracellular enzymes; active in carbohydrate and protein metabolism • Acts on myoneural junction, affecting neuromuscular irritability and contractility of cardiac and skeletal muscles • Affects peripheral vasodilation • Facilitates Na⁺ and K⁺ movement across all membranes • Influences Ca⁺⁺ levels	*Hypomagnesemia:* dizziness, confusion, seizures, tremor, leg and foot cramps, hyperirritability, arrhythmias, vasomotor changes, anorexia, and nausea *Hypermagnesemia:* drowsiness, lethargy, coma, arrhythmias, hypotension, vague neuromuscular changes (such as tremor), vague GI symptoms (such as nausea), and slow, weak pulse

Organs and hormones that maintain body fluid and electrolyte balance

Certain organs and hormones also help with regulating the body's delicate fluid and electrolye balance:

• The *pituitary gland* comprises an anterior and a posterior lobe. The posterior lobe releases antidiuretic hormone (ADH) into the circu-

lation. *ADH* increases water reabsorption into distal tubules and collecting ducts of the kidneys by inhibiting diuresis.
● The *adrenal glands* are responsible for the amount of sodium, potassium, and water that is retained or excreted. The adrenal glands secrete aldosterone, which acts as a volume regulator by saving sodium and releasing potassium to maintain normal sodium balance, thereby promoting normal water balance. An increase in aldosterone production can lead to excess sodium retention, and vice versa.
● The *kidneys* regulate body fluids and electrolyte excretion and secretion by selectively retaining or releasing electrolytes to maintain normal osmolarity and blood volume. In coordination with all regulating organs, the kidneys control the concentration of specific electrolytes, the osmolarity of body fluids, the volume of extracellular fluid, blood volume, and pH.
● The *parathyroid gland* releases parathyroid hormone, which regulates the calcium level. A decreased serum calcium level causes an increase in parathyroid secretion, resulting in increased reabsorption of calcium in the kidneys. An increase in the calcium level may cause the development of soft tissue calcifications.

Internal factors that regulate fluid and electrolyte balance
Internal factors also alter fluid and electrolyte status. These factors are discussed below:
● *Stretch receptors* are located in the atrial walls.
—An increase in volume stimulates the release of a hormone that increases sodium ion excretion, thereby increasing water excretion.
—An increase in volume also stimulates receptors that signal the brain to decrease sympathetic nervous system signals to the kidneys, thereby increasing urine output.
—An increase in volume stimulates receptors that signal the posterior pituitary gland to inhibit secretion of ADH, causing the kidneys to increase urine output.
—An increase in volume increases arterial blood pressure and stimulates baroceptors, which increase glomerular filtration rate (GFR), thus causing increased urine output.
● The hormone *atrial natriuretic peptide (ANP),* or atrial natriuretic factor (ANF), is released by the atria when atrial pressure increases. It responds by decreasing blood pressure and vascular volume.
● *Osmoreceptors* (receptors that detect change in osmotic pressure) in the hypothalamus, or thirst center, are excited by increased osmolarity of the extracellular fluid, causing the posterior pituitary gland to secrete ADH.
● *Stress* causes the kidneys to retain sodium and excrete potassium.
● *Thirst,* a result of an increase in osmotic pressure, causes fluid to leave the cells. This cellular dehydration stimulates osmoreceptors in the hypothalamus to transmit the sensation of thirst.

● *Insensible fluid loss,* also known as unconscious fluid loss, occurs via the skin and the lungs. The fluid lost through perspiration contains few electrolytes, thus constituting nearly pure water loss.

Acid-base balance

Electrolytes play a major role in everyday metabolism and physiologic functioning. One especially important function involves maintaining the body's acid-base balance — the proportion of carbonic acid (acid) to bicarbonate (base). The ratio of acid to base is normally 1:20.

An acid is a substance that releases hydrogen ions; a base is a substance that accepts hydrogen ions. Different electrolytes help maintain a normal acid-base environment by combining, competing for, or exchanging hydrogen ions. The concentration of hydrogen ions in the blood is measured by the pH. A balance must be maintained to keep the pH within a range of 7.35 to 7.45 to sustain life.

Although the pH provides much useful information about acid-base balance, this value alone is insufficient to determine the patient's true condition. A more thorough evaluation is made when the pH, arterial carbon dioxide ($PaCO_2$), and arterial bicarbonate (HCO_3^-) levels are evaluated together. Blood gas values obtained via an arterial puncture help evaluate all of these levels. Normal values include:

● pH: 7.35 to 7.45 (a pH of 7.35 or lower indicates acidity; 7.45 or higher indicates alkalinity, or basicity)

● $PaCO_2$: 35 to 45 mm Hg

● HCO_3^-: 22 to 26 mEq/liter.

The lungs and kidneys regulate acid-base changes to maintain balance. The lungs (respiratory component) control the amount of carbon dioxide, and thus carbonic acid, reacting rapidly to correct imbalances in approximately 1 to 2 minutes. The kidneys (metabolic component) control the bicarbonate level (HCO_3^-), reacting slowly over serveral hours to days to control balance. To maintain balance, an increase of acid necessitates an increase in bicarbonate, and vice versa.

Any alteration in normal acid-base balance can lead to medical problems if not quickly corrected.

● Conditions causing diminished respiration, such as sedation and retention of carbon dioxide, can result in *respiratory acidosis* (characterized by a pH below 7.35 and a $PaCO_2$ above 45 mm Hg).

● Conditions causing increased respiration, such as anxiety and hyperventilation, can result in *respiratory alkalosis* (indicated by a pH above 7.45 and a $PaCO_2$ below 35 mm Hg).

● Conditions causing an increase in fixed acids (ketoacidosis), such as renal failure and diabetes, that prevent bicarbonates from being produced cause *metabolic acidosis* (manifested by a pH below 7.35 and an HCO_3^- below 22 mEq/liter).

- Conditions causing an excess in bicarbonate production (such as decreased chloride levels from diuretics and vomiting, hypokalemia, and excess bicarbonate administration) can result in *metabolic alkalosis* (characterized by a pH above 7.45 and an HCO_3^- above 26 mEq/liter).

Other factors affecting fluid and electrolyte balance

Certain other factors involved in the control of fluid and electrolytes include:

- diseases or disorders that may disturb normal fluid and electrolyte balance, such as diabetes and colitis
- medications that may alter the normal balance of fluid and electrolytes, such as chemotherapeutic agents and diuretics
- treatments or procedures that may alter normal fluid and electrolyte balance, such as general surgery and nasogastric tube suctioning
- developmental age, social situation, psychological status, and spiritual and sociocultural beliefs.

FLUID AND ELECTROLYTE REPLACEMENT

Any patient with an illness or condition that prevents normal intake requires replacement of fluids through I.V. therapy. One general method of replacement is to provide 1 ml of free water for each replacement calorie, or 30 to 50 ml/kg body weight. Note that free water cannot be replaced intravenously as pure distilled water because distilled water would be drawn into the cell, causing cellular dilution, which allows the cell to swell and burst (a process called hemolysis). The addition of sodium and glucose to distilled water would make the solution isotonic, thereby preventing dilution of the cell components. Also, the glucose would add calories to the solution.

The following formula, which accounts for normal body fluid and electrolyte requirements, has been devised as the standard for I.V. replacement therapy:

Dextrose 5% in 25% solution of sodium chloride (each 100 ml contains 5 g dextrose and 225 mg sodium chloride in water for injection) plus 20 mEq/liter of potassium chloride to be infused at a daily rate based on the patient's fluid requirement per kilogram of body weight (generally, 30 to 50 ml/kg body weight).

However, each patient situation must be evaluated in light of the presence of disease or underlying conditions. For example, infusing a saline solution into a patient with congestive heart failure may be risky; the addition of sodium could cause water retention and further depress the patient's respiratory function. The composition of several different types of I.V. fluids used for fluid and electrolyte replacement is discussed in Chapter 2, I.V. Solutions. These I.V. fluids can be used in combination for fluid and electrolyte replacement, depending on the patient's individual condition.

FLUID BALANCE CHECKLIST

The following quick-reference checklist will help you assess your patient's fluid balance status. Remember that your priorities are to establish baseline vital signs and weight first and then monitor and record daily vital signs, weight, and fluid intake and output.

ASSESSMENT CHECKLIST	POTENTIAL PROBLEMS
Monitor weight	
☐ Loss of 5% or less	Mild dehydration
☐ Loss of 5% to 10%	Moderate dehydration
☐ Loss of more than 10%	Severe dehydration
☐ Gain of 5% or less	Mild overhydration
☐ Gain of 5% to 10%	Moderate overhydration
☐ Gain of more than 10%	Severe overhydration
Observe eyes	
☐ Dry conjunctiva	Fluid volume deficit
☐ Decreased tearing	
☐ Periorbital edema	
☐ Sunken eyes	
Observe mouth	
☐ Sticky, dry mucous membranes	Fluid volume deficit Sodium excess
☐ Increased viscosity of saliva	Sodium deficit
Observe lips	
☐ Dry, cracked	Fluid volume deficit
Observe tongue	
☐ Longitudinal furrows	Sodium deficit
Assess cardiovascular system	
☐ Increased pulse rate	Fluid volume deficit
☐ Decreased pulse rate	
☐ Decreased blood pressure	
☐ Narrowed pulse pressure	
☐ Bounding pulse	Fluid volume excess
☐ Jugular vein distention	
☐ Cardiac arrhythmias	Potassium deficit Magnesium deficit

(continued)

FLUID BALANCE: CHECKLIST *(continued)*

ASSESSMENT CHECKLIST	POTENTIAL PROBLEMS
Assess respiratory system	
☐ Moist crackles, rhonchi ☐ Increased respiratory rate ☐ Dyspnea ☐ Pulmonary edema	Fluid volume excess
☐ Shallow, slow breathing	Respiratory alkalosis with or without metabolic acidosis
☐ Deep, rapid breathing	Respiratory acidosis with or without metabolic alkalosis
Assess GI system	
☐ Absent bowel sounds ☐ Abdominal cramps	Potassium deficit Potassium excess
☐ Nausea, vomiting, and diarrhea ☐ Nausea and diarrhea ☐ Nausea, vomiting, and constipation	Magnesium excess Potassium excess Calcium excess
Assess renal system	
☐ Oliguria	Sodium deficit or excess Potassium excess
Observe extremities	
☐ Edema of dependent body parts	Fluid volume excess
Observe skin condition	
☐ Warm	Sodium excess
☐ Cold, clammy ☐ Poor skin turgor	Sodium deficit
☐ Warm, moist	Fluid volume excess
☐ Flushing	Magnesium deficit
Assess neurologic condition	
☐ Depressed central nervous system	Fluid volume deficit Electrolyte imbalance
☐ Increased intracranial pressure	Sodium deficit
☐ Positive Babinski's reflex	Magnesium deficit
☐ Disorientation or confusion	Fluid volume excess Acidosis or alkalosis Electrolyte imbalance
☐ Seizures	Calcium deficit Magnesium deficit

FLUID BALANCE: CHECKLIST *(continued)*	
ASSESSMENT CHECKLIST	*POTENTIAL PROBLEMS*
Observe musculoskeletal system	
☐ Muscle weakness	Potassium deficit Calcium excess
☐ Paralysis of flaccid muscles	Potassium excess
☐ Numbness in extremities	Potassium excess
☐ Hypertonicity (physical checks include positive Chvostek's sign[1], carpopedal[2] spasm)	Metabolic alkalosis Calcium deficit Magnesium deficit
☐ Muscle rigidity	Metabolic alkalosis
Monitor laboratory test results	
☐ Hematocrit elevation	Fluid volume excess or deficit Sodium excess
☐ Increased urine pH	Metabolic and respiratory alkalosis
☐ Decreased urine pH	Metabolic and respiratory acidosis
☐ Elevated blood urea nitrogen (BUN) and normal serum creatinine	Fluid volume deficit
Monitor urine specific gravity	
☐ Increased	Fluid volume deficit
☐ Decreased	Sodium deficit
☐ Increased red blood cells	Sodium excess or deficit Fluid volume excess

[1]Slight tapping of the facial nerve results in facial irritability.
[2]Spasms of the hands and feet.

Keep in mind that a 10% total fluid loss (about 4 liters) is considered serious. A 20% loss (about 8 liters) is usually fatal. Therefore, accurate assessment and documentation of the patient's total intake (including I.V. solutions, blood transfusions, and oral intake) and output (urination, vomitus, diarrhea, gastric secretions, bile, wound drainage, and drainage from fistulas) are essential during I.V. therapy. Fluid loss from fever and internal fluid shifts also must be considered. Daily weights should be obtained whenever possible. (See *Fluid Balance Checklist*, pages 15 to 17, for a sample worksheet to use for tracking your patient's fluid status.)

Laboratory results are also valuable in the early assessment of fluid balance (see *Laboratory Values and Their Significance*, page 18). However, note that normal values may vary among facilities.

LABORATORY VALUES AND THEIR SIGNIFICANCE

Laboratory test	Normal value	Significance
Serum osmolality: reflects total body hydration	280 to 295 mOsm/kg	• Increases in hydration • Decreases with water overload
Blood urea nitrogen: reflects the difference between rate of urea synthesis and excretion	8 to 20 mg/ 100 ml	• Increases with decreased renal blood flow or urine production, dehydration, some neoplasms, and certain antibiotics • Decreases in pregnancy, overhydration, severe hepatic damage, and malnutrition
Hematocrit: measures portion of blood volume occupied by red blood cells (RBCs)	Females: 38% to 46% Males: 43% to 51%	• Increases in dehydration • Decreases with low RBCs or normal hemoglobin and water overload
Creatinine (serum): measures products of muscle metabolism	0.2 to 1.5 mg/dl	• Elevated when 50% or more of the nephrons are destroyed
Urine osmolarity: measures number of particles per unit of water in urine	50 to 1,200 mOsm/liter (depends on the circulating titer of antidiuretic hormone and the rate of urinary solute excretion)	• Reflects changes in urine contents more accurately than specific gravity, depending on the previous state of hydration; urine osmolality should be 1½ times that of serum osmolality
Urine specific gravity: is inversely proportional to volume and measures urine concentration	1.010 to 1.030	• Increases with any condition causing hypoperfusion of kidneys, leading to oliguria (for example, shock or severe dehydration) • Decreases when tubules are unable to reabsorb water and concentrate urine
Urine pH: measures the acidity or alkalinity of urine	4.5 to 8.0	• Increases in metabolic and respiratory alkalosis, with magnesium-ammonium-phosphate stones or with certain urea-splitting infections (such as those caused by *Pseudomonas, Proteus,* and *Escherichia coli*) • Decreases with uric acid stones and with metabolic and respiratory acidosis • In renal acidosis, pH may be normal or slightly more acidic only when the plasma bicarbonate level is very low

To summarize, proper maintenance of the patient's fluid and electrolyte status involves performing a detailed patient evaluation. Baseline information on the patient's hydration status, a thorough review of all body systems, and a complete patient history are vital. This information, coupled with current laboratory values and an understanding of conditions that can lead to fluid and electrolyte imbalance, may mean the difference between life and death for your patient.

2 I.V. SOLUTIONS

I.V. solutions are generally used to replace fluid volume, restore fluid balance, supply calories, restore electrolyte balance, correct acid-base balance, and increase blood volume. Solutions vary in terms of their specific uses, contents, tonicity, compatibility with other solutions, and potential for complications.

Typically, I.V. solutions are composed of dextrose or sodium chloride, either alone or combined in different concentrations. Other electrolytes, such as calcium, magnesium, phosphate, acetate, or lactate, also may be included.

TYPES OF I.V. SOLUTIONS

I.V. solutions are classified by tonicity, or the osmotic pressure of the solution compared to normal serum plasma's concentration of solution and particles. Normal blood plasma has an osmolarity of approximately 290 mOsm/liter. A solution with approximately the same osmolarity as blood is called *isotonic*. A solution with an osmolarity of 340 mOsm/liter or more is considered *hypertonic*; one with 290 mOsm/liter or less is considered *hypotonic*. The tonicity of the I.V. solution can be determined easily by adding all the milliequivalents of the contents noted on the manufacturer's label.

Isotonic I.V. solutions are used to provide hydration in mildly dehydrated patients who have experienced a small fluid loss. They also may be used to expand fluid volume and maintain a "keep-vein-open" status for venous access. Common examples include dextrose 5% in water, normal saline (0.9% sodium chloride) solution, and lactated Ringer's solution.

Hypotonic I.V. solutions, those with a low solute content, are used to shift water into the intracellular compartment. They are commonly prescribed for severely dehydrated patients in whom dehydration is occurring at the cellular level. A common hypotonic solution is one-half normal saline (0.45% sodium chloride) solution. Sterile water is also hypotonic; however, it is never used as an I.V. infusion solution because it causes hemolysis, the destruction of red blood cells resulting from overhydration. Sterile water should never be used as an I.V. flush solution for the same reason.

Hypertonic I.V. solutions, those with a high solute content, are used to shift water out of the intracellular compartment. They are typically prescribed for patients with severe sodium deficit and water intoxication. Common examples include dextrose 10% to 70% in water and 3% to 5% sodium chloride solutions. These solutions must be administered very slowly to prevent circulatory overload and hypertension. (For more information, see *Administering I.V. Solutions,* page 21.)

ADMINISTERING I.V. SOLUTIONS

This chart lists some common examples of the three types of I.V. solutions—isotonic, hypotonic, and hypertonic—and provides key considerations for administering them.

Solution type	Examples	Nursing considerations
Isotonic • Osmolarity close to or equal to that of serum • Expands intravascular compartment only	• Lactated Ringer's solution (275 mOsm/liter) • Ringer's solution (275 mOsm/liter) • 0.9% sodium chloride solution (308 mOsm/liter) • Dextrose 5% in water (260 mOsm/liter)	• Closely monitor patient for signs of fluid overload because these solutions expand the intravascular compartment. • Do not give lactated Ringer's solution to a patient whose blood pH exceeds 7.5 because the liver converts lactate to bicarbonate. • Do not administer lactated Ringer's solution to a patient with liver disease because the patient will not be able to metabolize the lactate. • Avoid giving dextrose 5% in water to a patient who is at risk for increased intracranial pressure because it acts like a hypotonic solution (upon entering the body, the solution quickly metabolizes, leaving only water, a hypotonic fluid).
Hypotonic • Osmolarity lower than that of serum • Fluids and electrolytes shift out of the intravascular compartment, hydrating the intracellular and interstitial compartments	• 0.45% sodium chloride solution (154 mOsm/liter) • 0.33% sodium chloride solution (103 mOsm/liter) • Dextrose 2.5% in water (126 mOsm/liter)	• Administer these solutions cautiously because they can cause a sudden fluid shift from blood vessels into cells, causing cardiovascular collapse resulting from intravascular depletion and increased intracranial pressure (ICP) caused by fluid shift into brain cells. • Do not give hypotonic solutions to patients who are at risk for increased ICP resulting from cerebrovascular accident, head trauma, or neurosurgery. • Do not give hypotonic solutions to patients at risk for third-space fluid shifts (for example, patients with burns, trauma, or low serum protein levels caused by malnutrition or liver disease).

(continued)

ADMINISTERING I.V. SOLUTIONS *(continued)*		
Solution type	**Examples**	**Nursing considerations**
Hypertonic • Osmolarity higher than serum • Fluid and electrolytes drawn into the intravascular compartment from the intracellular and interstitial compartments	• Dextrose 5% in 0.45% sodium chloride solution (406 mOsm/liter) • Dextrose 5% in 0.9% sodium chloride solution (560 mOsm/liter) • Dextrose 5% and lactated Ringer's solution (575 mOsm/liter) • Dextrose 5% in 0.33% sodium chloride solution (355 mOsm/liter) • Dextrose 10% and water (505 mOsm/liter) • Dextrose 20% and water (1,010 mOsm/liter)	• Closely monitor the patient for signs of circulatory overload because these solutions greatly expand the intravascular compartment. • Do not administer these solutions to a patient with a condition that causes cellular dehydration (for example, diabetic ketoacidosis) because they pull fluid from the intracellular compartment. • Do not give these solutions to a patient with impaired heart or kidney function because the patient's system cannot handle the extra fluid.

Total parenteral nutrition (TPN) solutions, which are hypertonic, are infused into patients who cannot ingest food and fluids for a prolonged period, such as those who have lost adequate intestinal functioning. TPN replaces oral feedings, volume for volume, as well as any lost GI fluids and electrolytes. It contains approximately 20% glucose in 500 ml of water (this figure varies according to the patient) and 5% amino acids in 500 ml of water and supplies the patient with approximately 440 calories and 4 grams of nitrogen per liter. Because of the hypertonicity of the solution, central venous access is necessary. (TPN is discussed at length in Chapter 11, Parenteral Nutrition.)

DRUG COMPATIBILITY

Any nurse who administers I.V. therapy must be aware that certain medications may be incompatible with other medications or with the solutions in which they are mixed. Two types of incompatibilities, physical and chemical, can cause changes in I.V. solutions, either rendering the solutions inactive or potentiating their effect.

Physical incompatibilities may result from inadequate solubility or acid-base reactions. Signs of physical incompatibilities include precipitation (the settling out of small particles in a solution), color change, gas release, and cloudiness.

Chemical incompatibilities result from hydrolysis (chemical decomposition, which causes substances to split into simpler compounds) and from oxidation (the process of a substance combining with oxygen). Chemical incompatibilities are not obvious reactions; a breakdown in the chemical makeup of the substances is necessary for incompatibilities to occur.

Many factors can affect the compatibility of drugs and solutions, as indicated below.

Drug concentration

The concentration of one drug that comes in contact with another drug may result in the chemical instability of one or both drugs. For instance, if two medications are put into the same solution, they may not be chemically stable together. However, if the same two drugs are placed in separate bags of solution and administered together in piggyback fashion, they may remain stable.

pH of solution

The pH (degree of acidity or alkalinity) of an I.V. solution or its constituents may alter the effect and stability of drugs mixed in the solution:

- The pH of one drug may change when the drug is added to a solution of a different pH (for instance, antibiotics may be unstable in a solution with a pH of more than 8 or less than 4). The ideal pH for an I.V. solution is approximately 7.4; this is close to the pH of venous blood, which ranges from 7.35 to 7.45.
- If two drugs with different pH levels are mixed together in a solution, the resulting pH may inactivate the drugs or render them toxic to the patient.

In a patient with chemical phlebitis (explained in detail in Chapter 7, Complications), an investigation of the pH is warranted. A buffer solution of sodium bicarbonate, for example, may be added to help neutralize the pH of some solutions. This may prevent the phlebitis from worsening and make the infusion less painful for the patient. Check with the pharmacist about the possible effectiveness of sodium bicarbonate in altering the pH of a solution which cannot be tolerated before adding it to the solution or any other buffer added for such a patient.

Volume

Two drugs with high volumes may not be compatible; however, the same two drugs in smaller volumes may remain stable.

Length of time in contact

Two drugs mixed together and left in solution for a long period may result in incompatibility; however, the same two drugs administered quickly through the same catheter may remain stable because of their brief contact time.

Temperature

Some medications remain stable longer if refrigerated, whereas refrigeration for others may not be recommended.

Note: Remember that the potential for I.V. incompatibilities is very real and that incompatible solutions can cause serious adverse reactions for your patient. Always check for drug and solution compatibilities before administering any medication, regardless of whether it is given intravenously, intramuscularly, orally, or rectally. Drug compatibility charts are readily available from drug manufacturers and should be prominently displayed in all medication preparation areas.

POTENTIAL FOR COMPLICATIONS

Be aware that the administration of I.V. solutions can cause local or systemic complications for your patient. Local complications include:
- chemical phlebitis, vein irritation, or pain at the I.V. site (caused by solutions with a high or low pH or a high osmolarity, such as 40 mEq/liter of potassium chloride, phenytoin, and some antibiotics)
- venous spasm (caused by irritating drugs or fluids, infusion of fluids that are too cold, or very rapid flow rates of fluids at room temperature).

Systemic complications may include:
- circulatory overload (from a too-rapid flow rate or a miscalculation of the patient's fluid replacement needs)
- allergic reaction (from hypersensitivity to medications added to the solution).

SOLUTION PREPARATION

Each facility has its own system of obtaining and administering I.V. medications and solutions. No system is fail-proof. Since the development of the unit-dose delivery system, most I.V. medications have been distributed premixed by the manufacturer (for example, many commonly ordered medications, such as I.V. potassium solutions and continuous heparin infusions, are premixed by the manufacturer to save time). The safety and sterility of the solutions are the responsibility of the manufacturer, who must guarantee sterile admixtures as well as maintain sterile conditions when transporting the fluids.

However, nurses are responsible for double-checking the medication order and drug label before administering any premixed I.V. solution. Always read the medication bag carefully to ensure that it is the correct drug, given your patient's history and medical diagnosis, as well as the proper dosage. Many medication labels are similar in appearance, and errors often result from carelessness or not taking the time to double-check.

Pharmacies that prepare and distribute I.V. solutions usually use a computerized delivery system called an automated compounder for making the solutions. This is especially necessary when preparing TPN solutions that are specific to each patient's needs. Typically, the physician orders ingredients the patient requires, and the pharmacist prepares the solution quickly and accurately using the computerized delivery system.

In some cases, you will need to combine the appropriate drug with an I.V. solution at the patient's bedside before administering I.V. therapy, thereby guaranteeing a fresh admixture. This allows you to see the medication in the bottle before adding it to the solution to ensure that the proper medication is being administered to the patient.

INITIATING THERAPY
Regardless of who prepares the solution, as a nurse, you are responsible for verifying the medication label against physician's orders, using the proper diluent (or verifying that the correct diluent was used in a premixed solution), checking the additives, ensuring drug compatibility, and avoiding the administration of blood products with any drugs. Also be sure to inspect the solution for cloudiness, discoloration, and precipitation. Never cut corners. If you have any questions or doubts about the solution, consult the pharmacist.

The Intravenous Nurses Society recommends the following when initiating I.V. therapy:
● Ascertain the physician's order.
● Be sure that the physician's orders for I.V. therapy are written and signed. Any verbal orders should be recorded by a registered nurse and signed by the physician within 24 hours.
● Follow the nursing process (assessment, diagnosis, planning, implemention, and evaluation) to determine the appropriateness of the medical order in terms of the patient's needs.
● Identify the patient.
● Explain the procedure, the specific therapy, and any special considerations to the patient. Remember, the patient has the right to refuse therapy.
● Collect and assemble appropriate equipment (see Chapter 3, I.V. Equipment), and ensure asepsis.
● If you have any doubt about the physician's orders (verbal or written), clarify the order before administering the medication. Failure to do so could result in a malpractice lawsuit.

Always remember the five rights of medication administration—time, dose, route, medication, and patient—when providing I.V. therapy to any patient. Be sure that the correct patient receives the correct medication, in the correct dose, at the correct time, via the correct route. Also remember that the patient has the right to refuse treatment as well as the right to information about his or her condition and treatment.

3

I.V. EQUIPMENT

Part of your responsibility in providing I.V. therapy involves being able to identify, assemble, and maintain I.V. equipment. This equipment includes venous access devices (needles and cannulas), protective devices (needle shields and other safety devices), I.V. tubing and accessories (ports, valves, and filters), dressings, and pumps.

VENOUS ACCESS DEVICES

I.V. fluids can be delivered either peripherally or centrally, depending on the patient's condition and needs. Peripheral venous access devices, such as scalp-vein needles and over-the-needle cannulas, are typically used for short-term (less than 4 weeks) or intermittent I.V. therapy. Peripheral venous therapy involves the administration of fluid through a vein in the arm or hand (or occasionally in a leg or foot).

Central venous devices allow the administration of fluid through a central vein, such as the right or left subclavian vein or the internal or external jugular vein. Generally, the device is left in place for a long time. In some cases, central venous devices are surgically implanted in a subcutaneous pocket for use in long-term (months to years) therapy. (For more specific information about the types of venous access devices, see *Peripheral Venous Access Devices,* pages 28 and 29, and *Central Venous Catheters,* pages 30 to 32.

The purpose of any device used in I.V. therapy is to supply the patient with needed fluids, medications, blood, or blood by-products. Sometimes, the design of the device can be more hazardous than helpful. A well-designed catheter can decrease the risk of infection by limiting skin or vein trauma. When selecting a venous access device, consider the following factors:

- *Who is the patient?* Some designs are better suited for young or elderly patients, who may benefit from smaller lengths and gauges, and softer materials, such as Vialon.
- *How long will the cannula remain in place?* Catheters left in place longer than 72 hours are associated with a higher risk of complications. Promoting hemodilution, or the amount of blood flow around the catheter, is important. Again, a smaller and softer catheter is better.
- *What will be infused through the cannula?* Sometimes a larger gauge may be necessary to infuse more viscous liquids, such as blood. Promoting hemodilution by using smaller, softer catheters is important.
- *What material is the cannula made of?* The over-the-needle catheter, the most commonly used device, is available in a variety of materials

(Text continues on page 32.)

PERIPHERAL VENOUS ACCESS DEVICES

The chart below describes the most commonly used venous access devices for peripheral I.V. therapy.

Device	Description	Advantages and disadvantages
Scalp-vein needle (SVN; also called winged-tip or butterfly) *Purpose:* Used for short-term therapy for cooperative patients 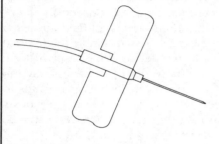	• Stainless-steel needle appropriate for short-term therapy. • Available in odd-numbered gauges. • Manufactured with extension tubing.	*Advantages* • Excellent for one-time I.V. medication infusion, for blood withdrawal, and for patients allergic to nylon or Teflon. • Wings allow for secure taping. • Attached extension allows tubing to be changed without site manipulation and cross-contamination. • Bleedback is easy to control with syringe or manufacturer's cap on hub of extension tubing or by pinching extension tubing. • Decreases nurse's exposure to patient's blood. *Disadvantages* • Needle increases risk of infiltration. • Not recommended for use in flexor areas or in active children. • Requires a vein long and straight enough for length of needle. • Needle is not flexible. • Repuncture by contaminated needle is possible if it is dislodged.
Over-the-needle catheters *Purpose:* Designed to provide long-term therapy for active or agitated patients. **Type A** 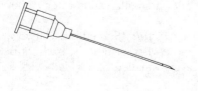	• Clear plastic catheter joins square metal hub with little difference in size. • Available in even-numbered gauges and various lengths. • Catheter tip is tapered only slightly.	*Advantages* • Easy to insert; they glide into the skin without drag. *Disadvantages* • Square hub is difficult to secure. • Metal junction between catheter and metal hub can tear or further penetrate the skin, causing pain and increasing the risk of infection. • Long, inflexible stylet increases risk of accidental puncture after its removal from catheter. • Catheter is not tapered enough to prevent peelback. • Uncomfortable for many patients. • Pressure marks are common. • Can accidentally dislodge because hub is not flat. • Bleedback is difficult to control (applying pressure on vein above catheter tip may help).

PERIPHERAL VENOUS ACCESS DEVICES *(continued)*		
Device	**Description**	**Advantages and disadvantages**
Type B	• Plastic hub joins an obviously different-sized catheter.	*Advantages* • Enlargement of insertion site is possible, but not likely. • Catheter tip is tapered to prevent peelback. • Radiopaque feature makes X-ray detection easy. *Disadvantages* • Catheter is difficult to secure because of hub shape, which increases risk of mechanical phlebitis. • Long, inflexible stylet increases risk of accidental puncture after its removal from cannula. • Easy to pull out accidentally because catheter hub is raised on skin and can get caught on clothing or sheets. • Shape of hub limits comfort. • Catheter may cause pressure marks. • Bleedback is difficult to control (applying pressure to vein above catheter tip is the only option).
Type C	• Winged design resembles SVN. • Manufactured with extension tubing and a Y port, which ensures virtually bloodless venipuncture. • Catheter tip is well-tapered. • Less of a "pop" is felt by nurse and patient as a result of tapered tip design. • Now available in sheathing design.	*Advantages* • Wings allow for secure taping. • If pulled out accidentally, repuncture is impossible because no needle remains. • Long, flexible stylet makes accidental puncture after its removal from catheter and cross-contamination unlikely. • Radiopaque feature makes X-ray detection easy. • Excellent design helps prevent mechanical and bacterial phlebitis and ensures patient comfort. • Elimination of the "pop" sensation decreases pain on insertion. • Bleedback is easy to control because of extension tubing; pinching tubing prevents spillage of bleedback (pressure at catheter tip is another bleedback control method). *Disadvantages* • Tends to be slightly more expensive than straight-stylet design catheters.

CENTRAL VENOUS CATHETERS

Central venous (CV) catheters differ in their design, construction, and indications. The following chart provides a description of each type along with advantages, diadvantages, and nursing considerations for some of the most commonly used CV catheters.

Catheter	Description and indications	Advantages and disadvantages	Nursing considerations
Short-term multiple-lumen catheter	• Polyvinyl chloride (PVC) or polyurethene construction with two, three, or four lumens located at ¾" (2 cm) intervals; lumen gauges vary. • Used for short-term CV access, typically for patient with limited insertion sites who requires multiple infusions.	*Advantages* • Easily inserted at bedside. • Easily removed. • Stiffness aids central. venous pressure (CVP) monitoring. • Allows infusion of multiple solutions through the same catheter—even incompatible solutions. *Disadvantages* • Limited functions. • PVC is thrombogenic. • PVC irritates inner layer of vessel. • Needles need to be changed every 3 to 7 days.	• Minimize patient motion. • Assess frequently for signs of infection and clot formation. • Be familiar with gauge and purpose of each lumen. • Use the same lumen for the same task (for example, administering total parenteral nutrition [TPN] or drawing or blood samples).
Groshong catheter	• Silicone rubber construction, approximately 35" (88.9 cm) long. • Has closed end with pressure-sensitive two-way valve and a Dacron cuff; available with one or two lumens. • Used for long-term CV access; suitable for patient with heparin allergy.	*Advantages* • Less thrombogenic. • Pressure-sensitive two-way valve eliminates need for frequent heparin flushes. • Dacron cuff anchors catheter and prevents bacterial migration. *Disadvantages* • Requires surgical insertion. • Tears and kinks easily. • Blunt end makes it difficult to clear substances from tip.	• Provide dressing care for surgical sites after insertion. • Handle catheter gently. • Check external portion frequently for kinks or leaks (repair kit is available). • Remember to flush with enough saline solution to clear catheter, especially after withdrawing or administering blood.

CENTRAL VENOUS CATHETERS (continued)

Catheter	Description and indications	Advantages and disadvantages	Nursing considerations
Hickman catheter	• Silicone rubber construction, approximately 35" long. • Has open end with clamp; Dacron cuff is located 11¾" (30 cm) from hub; available with one or multiple lumens. • Used for long-term CV access, including home therapy.	*Advantages* • Less thrombogenic. • Dacron cuff prevents excess motion and organism migration. • Clamps eliminate need for Valsalva maneuver. *Disadvantages* • Requires surgical insertion. • Has an open end. • Requires removal by physician. • Tears and kinks easily.	• Provide dressing care for surgical sites after insertion. • Handle catheter gently. • Observe frequently for kinks or tears (repair kit is available). • Clamp catheter any time it becomes disconnected or open, using a nonserrated clamp.
Broviac catheter	• Identical to Hickman, except it has a smaller inner lumen. • Used for long-term CV access; suitable for patient with small central vessels (especially pediatric and elderly patients).	*Advantages* • Smaller lumen ensures better comfort. *Disadvantages* • Limited use because of smaller lumen. • Has only one lumen.	• Follow facility's policy for drawing or administering blood or blood products.
Hickman-Broviac catheter	• Includes Hickman and Broviac units in one catheter. • Used for long-term CV access, especially for patient who require multiple-lumen infusions.	*Advantages* • Double-lumen Hickman unit allows sampling and administration of blood. • Broviac lumen allows delivery of I.V. fluids, including TPN. *Disadvantages* • Requires surgical insertion. • Has an open end. • Requires removal by physician. • Tears and kinks easily.	• Know purpose and function of each lumen. • Label lumens to prevent confusion.

(continued)

CENTRAL VENOUS CATHETERS *(continued)*

Catheter	Description and indications	Advantages and disadvantages	Nursing considerations
Peripherally inserted central catheter (PICC) and midline catheter	• Silicone rubber construction. • PICC is 20" to 24" (51 to 61 cm) long; midline catheter is 6" to 8" (15 to 20 cm) long. • Available in 16G, 18G, and 20G sizes. • Used for long-term CV access, especially in patients with poor central access, those at risk for complications from central insertion, and those who need CV access but must undergo head and neck surgery.	*Advantages* • Peripherally inserted. • Easily inserted at bedside with minimal complications. • May be inserted by qualified RN in some states. *Disadvantages* • Catheter may occlude smaller peripheral vessels. • May be difficult to keep immobile, increasing the risk for malpositioning. • Has only one lumen. • Provides a long path to CV circulation.	• Check frequently for signs of phlebitis and thrombus formation. • Insert catheter above the antecubital fossa. • Use armboard, if necessary, to immobilize catheter. • Be aware that catheter may alter CVP measurements.

(such as Teflon, Vialon, Aquavene, Silastic, and polyurethane). Vialon and Teflon, the oldest type of over-the-needle catheter, are probably the most commonly used. However, Teflon is less pliable than the other materials and tends to cause more trauma to the intima layer (the inner layer of the vein, which is only one cell layer thick and easily destroyed). Also, because the material cannot be tapered to a thin edge, Teflon does not readily penetrate the skin, which results in peelback, or splitting, of the catheter at the tip. The newer materials generally are more vein-friendly.

Stainless steel needles, the oldest style of venous access device on the market, are not widely used except when drawing blood and administering short-term I.V. therapy; occasionally, they are used for patients who are allergic to the other types of catheter materials. Stainless steel catheters generally are not used for continuous I.V. therapy because the needle is left in place and the chances of infiltration are high.

The ideal catheter

Nurses seldom have a voice in determining which needles and catheters their facility stocks. However, being aware of the pros and cons of various designs may help you to influence purchasing decisions. An ideally designed catheter should have the following features:

- easy to insert (the design of the tip is important). A thin-walled tapered tip will glide more smoothly through the skin and vein wall and cause less trauma to the intima layer of the vein.
- easy to secure with tape (check the hub design). The flatter the hub, the more comfortable it will be for the patient. Round hubs without wings are more difficult to secure and more uncomfortable for the patient. Round hubs also leave pressure grooves in the skin and have been known to tear thin skin.
- allow control of flashback (blood return). Flashback is essential in verifying correct catheter placement. The ideal catheter should provide user control over flashback.

The following design problems can cause complications:

- easy dislodgment of cannula (will disrupt therapy and may accidentally stick the patient or nurse)
- excessive cannula movement within vein (can injure the vein)
- bulky hub (may injure the patient's skin)
- thickly tapered cannula tip (may fray or split, injuring the patient's tunica intima).

Regardless of the type of I.V. therapy, the gauge and length of the catheter must always be considered. According to Intravenous Nurses Society (INS) standards, always use the smallest gauge and length of catheter that will safely infuse the ordered therapy (for general I.V. therapy, a 22-gauge [22G] catheter is commonly used). Following this standard will promote hemodilution and decrease vein trauma, thereby promoting healthy veins.

Protective vascular devices

Since the onset of acquired immunodeficiency syndrome (AIDS), medical professionals have been greatly concerned about the potential hazards involved in the administration of I.V. therapy. All catheters will do the job, but some are better than others at accessing veins, preventing vein trauma, and protecting both the patient and the health care worker from unnecessary needlesticks and exposure to blood. Some older equipment offer added safety features, whereas most newer equipment include built-in protective features.

The decision of whether to continue using older equipment or to invest in newer equipment in many cases rests with the facility and, to a large degree, indirectly rests with the nurses and other health care workers who will be using the equipment. Each facility must evaluate its needs and the various venous access systems carefully to choose the most effective system. Keep in mind, though, that drastic changes in procedures and equipment may lead to disaster. If the addition of too many pieces of equipment or parts that are difficult to assemble proves cumbersome to nurses, the equipment will not be used; nurses will find ways to adapt the new equipment to older parts, thereby neglecting the safety features and wasting the facility's money.

For over a decade, such equipment as the Angioset and the Intima (both available with a Y-site adapter), have provided over-the-needle catheters with added safety features to prevent needlesticks and to allow control of flashback. Although not classified as protective devices or part of a "needleless system," these devices are uniquely designed to be beneficial to all types of patients and all health care workers. Similar catheters that are classified as protective devices are designed with a sheathing system for further protection.

Several new devices have been developed to guard specifically against needlesticks and blood exposure:

● shielded or recessed needle. This consists of a needle encased in a plastic housing that fits over a latex port. However, because of the presence of the needle, disposal containers must still be used. Also, the availability of a latex port allows nurses to bypass the shield, thereby decreasing the chance for compliance with use of this safety feature.

● needleless system. Probably the most expensive protective device; it necessitates the replacement of all existing I.V. tubing and syringes and substitution of plastic cannulas for needles. Latex ports are still present and needles can theoretically be used, so compliance is not guaranteed. However, the cost of needle disposal is greatly reduced.

● blunted needle. Probably the least expensive option, but noncompliance is possible due to the presence of a latex port. Proper needle disposal is still required.

● valve system. This replaces ports with valves that cannot be accessed with a needle. Like the needleless system, the valve system may cost a little more; however, it can be adapted to most systems already being used. The valve may be placed on the end of all cannula hubs. Compliance with this system is guaranteed.

I.V. SETUPS
Each I.V. set includes tubing, a drip system, a flow regulator, ports, valves, adapters, and, possibly, filters (for an illustration of a basic I.V. setup, see *Basic I.V. Set,* page 35). The following information highlights features common to most I.V. administration sets.

I.V. infusion tubing
I.V. infusion tubing is available in both vented and unvented forms to ensure proper flow of fluids. Vented tubing is used with I.V. bottles that have no inherent venting system. Unvented tubing is used with solution bags and vented bottles. Some delivery systems (such as I.V.

BASIC I.V. SET

A basic I.V. set, which is used to administer most I.V. solutions, consists of a piercing spike, a drop orifice, a drip chamber, one or more Y-site injection ports, a roller clamp, and a luer-lock adapter or needle adapter. Basic sets range from 70″ to 110″ (178 to 279 cm) long and can be vented or unvented. The illustration below shows a typical vented set with a backcheck valve and three Y-site injection ports.

BASIC SET   **ADD-A-LINE SET**

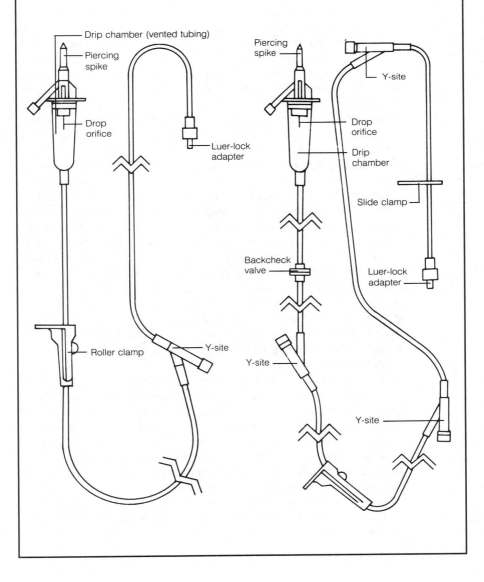

pumps, controllers, and other electronic delivery systems) require tubing specifically designed for that particular machine. *Note:* For standardization and cost-effectiveness, facilities typically stock only one type of tubing. The vented set functions nicely for both bottles and bags; however, the nonvented ones can be used for I.V. bags only.

The I.V. tubing also controls the flow rate. Macrodrip (also called maxidrip) tubing delivers 10, 15, or 20 drops/ml. Microdrip (also called minidrip) tubing delivers 60 drops/ml. Two factors influence which type of I.V. tubing is used for certain rates: the accurate counting of drops and movement through the catheter (which prevents clotting resulting from blood backing up in the tubing). Using microdrip tubing for I.V. rates over 75 ml/hour requires counting more than 75 gtts/minute; it is difficult to ensure accurate counting in this situation. Using macrodrip tubing for I.V. rates less than 50 ml/hour would result in less than 10 gtts/minute being infused; this may lead to blood backing up in the tubing and a clotted I.V. cannula as well as possible clotting of the system because too much time will elapse between drops, thus slowing the movement of the solution through the catheter. Therefore, use microdrip tubing for rates < 50 ml/hour and macrodrip tubing for rates > 75 ml/hour. Use either for rates of 50 to 75 ml/hour.

I.V. tubing must be changed regularly to prevent in-line bacteremia (see Chapter 1, Introduction to I.V. Therapy, for more information on infection control). I.V. administration sets should be changed at least every 72 hours; ideally, the changing of the set should be done the same time a new container is started. However, tubing should be changed every 24 hours whenever blood products or lipid emulsions are administered, or when infusion-related septicemia is suspected. These timetables reflect common practice among facilities; however, INS recommends changing the I.V. tubing as follows:

- continuous I.V. infusion set — every 48 hours
- intermittent infusion set — every 24 hours
- total parenteral nutrition infusion set — every 24 hours
- blood administration set — after every unit of blood
- lipid infusion set — after every bottle
- pressure monitoring tubing set — every 48 hours.

Changing the tubing and accessory equipment every 24 to 72 hours probably provides the best protection against infection caused by contamination. More frequent tubing changes should be considered when a patient receives numerous piggyback and I.V. push medications. However, whenever a system is interrupted, bacteria can be introduced through the tubing ports. Numerous port penetrations also increase the chance of infusion-related septicemia.

A logical patient-oriented approach to tubing change helps ensure that each patient's I.V. system best suits his or her needs. This involves assessing each situation and adjusting the routine accordingly. Make one shift responsible for all routine tubing changes to ensure that basics are performed. Enforce labeling the I.V. set and documenting changes to ensure that I.V. sets are changed appropriately.

Infusion ports

Infusion ports allow additional solutions to be given through the main I.V. line. The upper port, or piggyback port, is reserved for intermittent drug administration. To ensure proper flow rate, use shorter tubing with the solution to be piggybacked. Keeping the tubing short prevents the formation of loops, which could inhibit the flow rate of the piggyback solution.

The secondary port, or lower Y-site, is reserved for intermittent or simultaneous drug administration. Although piggybacks with longer tubing may be infused in the secondary port, this practice generally is not recommended because gravity can interrupt the flow, and the extra tubing can be awkward for the ambulatory patient.

The upper port of some I.V. tubing includes a backcheck valve, which prevents a piggyback solution from backing up into the main I.V. solution. Main I.V. solutions will not run when the piggyback solution is running via the upper infusion port. The secondary port has no backcheck valve; I.V. solutions and piggybacks may run simultaneously through this port.

Whatever type of tubing you use, always remember to read the manufacturer's package for instructions on how to use the set. All I.V. tubings are not alike. Some include a backcheck valve; others do not. Some have two medication ports; others have none. Some I.V. sets have filters; others do not. Be sure that the set you use is appropriate for the type of I.V. therapy prescribed for your patient. Choosing and opening the wrong setup can be costly, both for the patient and for the facility. Also, each tubing change predisposes the patient to sepsis.

Flow regulators

Flow regulators help to ensure accurate delivery of I.V. fluids by delivering a specific number of milliliters of solution per hour.

Clamps

Clamps regulate the flow of the I.V. solution. The roller clamp and screw clamp increase or decrease the flow. The slide clamp will only stop and start the flow.

Flow-control add-on devices

The STAT 2, STAT2 Pumpette, and Dial-A-Flo are control devices that can be attached to the I.V. tubing to set a specific flow rate of milliliters per hour. They attach to the end of I.V. tubing with the roller clamp wide open. The rate is regulated by the controlling device.

The STAT 2 and Dial-A-Flo are gravity-flow devices. The I.V. solution must be at least 3 feet above the level of the heart for adequate flow.

Changes in gravity or patient position can stop or slow the rate of flow. The STAT 2 Pumpette is attached in the same manner as the STAT 2 and Dial-A-Flo, but it is not a gravity-flow device. It contains a small pumpette that maintains the rate when the level of gravity is changed, making its control of the flow rate more reliable.

Use all add-on flow control devices carefully, and observe for proper flow rate frequently. These devices are a simple means of monitoring the rate; however, as with any equipment that is attached to I.V. tubing, the potential for bacteria to enter the I.V. system via the connections exists. Maintain all I.V. tubing and add-on devices using aseptic technique. For more precise monitoring, use electronic devices.

Volume-control fluid chambers
Volume-control fluid chambers provide more delicate control. The Soluset or Buretrol sets are examples of volume-control fluid chambers that deliver small doses of medication over an extended period. Volume-control sets provide excellent protection against fluid and medication overload and deliver a more titrated volume. They contain a fluid chamber to measure the volume of the dose, and a drip chamber below to measure the flow rate. Volume-control I.V. sets should be used with all patients on fluid restriction and with all pediatric patients.

I.V. filters
I.V. filters help protect the patient from hazardous microorganisms and debris that may collect in the I.V. solution. Filters may be added to any infusion tubing that does not contain its own in-line filter. However, keep in mind that contamination is still possible despite taking precautions to ensure a sterile solution.

Particulate matter that can be found in admixtures includes:
- dissolved impurities in water, such as detergents, proteins, and polysaccharides
- salt from soil, rocks, pipes, and tanks
- microorganisms that, if alive, will multiply in the bloodstream or, if dead, will enter the tissue and cause a sterile abscess
- particles of metal, lint, asbestos, rubber, cotton, dust, or glass
- undissolved drugs, powders, or crystals
- precipitates from incompatible mixtures.

Standard sterile I.V. solutions may not need to be filtered; however, if adding a medication to an I.V. line requires breaking an ampule or invading a rubber stopper, a filtered needle (needle with a 0.45-micron filter inside it) should be used and a final filter should be added to the I.V. tubing.

Consider using a filtered needle attached to a syringe or a filter attached to I.V. tubing to prevent introduction of impurities when:
- combining an additive with an I.V. solution.
- pushing medications into ports along the I.V. tubing (use filtered needles).

- caring for a patient who is especially susceptible to phlebitis or infection (INS recommends using 0.22-micron air-eliminating filters to effectively screen bacteria, thereby reducing the risk of I.V.-related sepsis). Always remember to change to a new filtered needle or a regular needle when injecting the drawn solution into the bag or patient. It is possible to flush out some or all of the collected debris.

Three basic types of filters are available:

- depth filters, which remove a percentage of particulate matter
- membrane filters with calculated pore sizes that vary in rating (for example, 0.22-micron, 0.45-micron, 1.0-micron, 1.2-microns, 5.0-microns, and 20.0-microns). These filters are used to remove air, undissolved drug particles, bacteria, and fungi.
- screen filters with ratings of 40.0-microns, 80.0-microns, and 170.0-microns. These filters are used to remove clots and cell debris.

The filter size indicates which particles can pass through the filter membrane. Filters are capable of removing particulate matter, clots, air, cell debris, undissolved drug particles, bacteria, and fungi as long as the filter size is appropriate. However, no filter is designed to remove viruses. Keep in mind that, when a pump is used, the filter also must be able to withstand the pressure generated by the pump (pounds per square inch [psi]).

When drawing up medication for intramuscular administration, a filtered needle may be beneficial in eliminating particulate matter from the solution. Be sure to change to a regular needle when injecting medication into a patient.

Keep in mind that the terminal in-line 0.22- or 0.45-micron membrane filters may reduce contamination and offer the patient the most complete protection. Final filters, placed at the end of the continuous fluid or closest to the patient, are probably the most beneficial and cost-effective (instead of in-line filters). The filter must be changed routinely and be observed for proper function. More frequent changes may be necessary if the filter becomes blocked. This requires added system manipulation, allowing a greater potential for contamination. Furthermore, filters are expensive and they have not been shown to consistently reduce morbidity associated with infusion therapy. So use filters wisely and efficiently.

Other I.V. accessories

Accessories for I.V. needles and cannulas may improve venous access, increase patient comfort and tolerance, and prevent complications. For more information, see *Accessory Equipment,* page 40. Keep in mind that added equipment means added cost, so choose accessories wisely. Also remember that each connection point provides a port of entry for bacteria.

ACCESSORY EQUIPMENT

Description	Advantages	Disadvantages
PRN adapters • May have luer-lock or luer-slip connection. • Also called catheter plug. 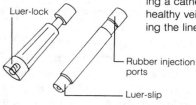	• Converts continuous I.V. infusion to an intermittent device by inserting plug into cannula hub. • Less costly than removing a catheter from a healthy vein and restarting the line.	• Can separate at hub or plug junction, allowing bacteria to enter.
T port • Helps prevent site manipulation. 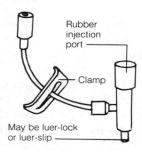	• Provides a small extension for easy tubing change and an extra port close to the cannula for I.V. push medications. • Excellent addition to help secure jugular and subclavian I.V. lines. • Useful when added to Huber needles to clamp line between syringes when withdrawing blood or infusing I.V. push medications via an Infuse-A-Port.	• Adds to overall cost. • Extra junction allows for accidental separation and entrance of bacteria.
Extension tubings • Added to exisiting tubing for more length and extra ports. • May or may not have a clamp on tubing. 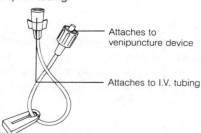	• Adds length to I.V. line for active patients. • Aids in tubing change without site manipulation.	• Adds to overall cost. • Adds sites for bacteria to enter the system.

Image labels:
- Luer-lock
- Rubber injection ports
- Luer-slip
- Rubber injection port
- Clamp
- May be luer-lock or luer-slip
- Attaches to venipuncture device
- Attaches to I.V. tubing

INTERMITTENT INFUSION DEVICES

Intermittent infusion devices, commonly called I.V. locks or heparin locks, are used to infuse occasional medications and to draw or infuse blood. Any I.V. catheter, even a central venous access device, can be converted to an intermittent infusion device by removing the tubing and inserting a catheter plug (PRN adapter). Because fluid does not flow continuously through an intermittent infusion device, special precautions must be taken to prevent blood clotting in the cannula. Some facilities choose to heparinize their I.V. locks to prevent clot formation in the cannula (this is why they are also called heparin locks). The heparinization procedure for a peripheral I.V. lock, commonly known as SASH, involves the following steps:

- *Saline.* Inject 2 to 5 ml of normal saline solution (0.9% sodium chloride) into the cannula to flush the previously injected solution and prevent mixing medications.
- *Antibiotic or Admixture.* Perform the required procedure, such as infusing the piggyback medication or withdrawing blood. If blood is drawn, the first 3 to 5 ml will be diluted. Discard this and withdraw another sample.
- *Saline.* Flush the cannula again with 2 to 5 ml of normal saline solution.
- *Heparin flush.* Inject 1 to 5 ml of diluted heparin solution (typically 100 units) into the catheter to prevent thrombus formation in the catheter and at its tip.

Note: the amount of saline should be two to four times the amount the cannula holds. Remember that *more is better.* Do not be afraid of using too much saline when flushing.

Ongoing studies are attempting to determine whether flushing with normal saline solution alone is sufficient to maintain patency in heparin locks. This would eliminate the need to expose the patient to routine heparinization. Depending on the results of these studies, flushing may become routine practice in the future. A recent study indicated that approximately 60% of the facilities surveyed still heparinize their peripheral intermittent I.V. infusion systems.

If saline alone is used to ensure patency and prevent bacteria from entering your peripheral intermittent infusion devices, be sure to exit the PRN adapter with positive pressure. This means that you will push saline until the syringe is almost empty and pull out of the PRN adapter while still pushing. If you stop pushing and then remove the needle from the PRN adapter, negative pressure is created. This pulls blood back into the catheter, making it more likely to clot in the cannula.

Keep in mind the following points when administering I.V. solutions:

- When you inject medication into an intermittent infusion device, a small amount will remain in the catheter. Flushing the catheter with normal saline solution after the medication is infused will ensure that the patient receives the entire dose ordered.

- When you discontinue the lock after injecting medication, flush the catheter with normal saline solution before removing it. This procedure will remove all irritating or vesicant solution from the catheter tip. Even the smallest amount of some medications can cause severe irritation or tissue damage.
- Although only 1 to 2 ml (or less) of solution may remain in the catheter after an injection, precipitation can still result if the solution is not compatible with the next medication. Using a saline flush will prevent medications from mixing in the catheter.

An I.V. lock (that is, an intermittent infusion) administered via a central line should be heparinized to maintain patency and to prevent clot formation. Positive-pressure instillation of heparin is necessary to prevent the blood from backing up into the cannula after flushing.

The amount of sodium chloride and heparin used is dictated by an individual facility's policy and procedures. However, the length of the cannula hub and the distance between the point of injection and the canulla hub should be taken into consideration. Some institutions have adopted this particular standard flushing procedure for all central lines:

S — 10 ml saline

A — administer medication

S — 10 ml saline

H — 5 ml of 10 units/ml heparin.

Care for the intermittent infusion device as you would any venous access device. Dressing care, site care, and site rotations should be done as if I.V. solution were running through the catheter. Check the PRN adapter for leakage from the port caused by continuous needle penetration, and change the adapter when necessary. A port that has lost integrity will leak. This is no longer a closed system, and bacteria can enter. Also, the probability of losing positive pressure and allowing blood to back up and clot in the catheter increases.

CENTRAL VENOUS ACCESS DEVICES

Central venous (CV) devices are used for long-term I.V. therapy that may be required over weeks, months, or even years. Such devices allow access to a central vein for the administration of a large volume of fluid or for hypertonic solutions, caustic drugs, or total parenteral nutrition solutions. CV access also may be used when the patient has inaccessible peripheral veins or requires I.V. therapy at home. Common uses include chemotherapy infusion, multiple I.V. infusions, frequent blood withdrawal, and the administration of blood and blood products.

Most CV catheters are made of polyvinyl chloride (PVC), Teflon, polyurethane, or silicone. Silicone is the most vein-friendly because it is soft and pliable and reportedly has the lowest incidence of thrombus formation. All catheters, whether peripheral or central, should be radiopaque in case an X-ray is needed to locate the catheter within the venous system.

Triple-lumen CV cannulas

The triple-lumen CV catheter, formerly known as a subclavian line, is commonly used for critical care patients and those requiring emergency central venous access, such as in cardiac arrest. Placement is done by a physician, who inserts the cannula into the superior vena cava, through the subclavian vein or the internal or external jugular vein, with the tip positioned just before the right atrium. The catheter is then sutured in place. If a catheter placed beyond the axilla is used for any reason other than isotonic fluid administration, an X-ray is taken to verify tip placement. A CV catheter also may be used for femoral insertion.

Until the late 1980s, triple-lumen catheters were rarely used. The traditional subclavian line, which contains only one lumen, was used until then, and any triple-lumen device theoretically carried three times the risk for causing sepsis. However, because patients who were seriously ill enough for a central line typically needed more than one lumen, the demand for more lines (and more lumens) literally changed the name of the subclavian line to the triple-lumen catheter.

Each lumen terminates at various points along the catheter to permit blood withdrawal, I.V. fluid infusion, I.V. medication administration, and blood transfusions through one catheter. The exit ports are approximately ¾" (2 cm) apart, and hemodilution decreases the amount of mixing from three simultaneous infusions.

Care for a triple-lumen catheter is much the same as for any central venous device. According to INS, these catheters should remain in place for 3 to 10 days. All central lines should be clamped while changing tubing or PRN adapters. It is possible for the patient to suffer air embolism if air is allowed to enter the catheter.

Midline catheters and peripherally inserted central catheters (PICCs)

Midline catheters and PICCs are peripherally inserted through the antecubital fossa. The difference between the two is where the tip terminates in the vasculature. They are both soft, silastic catheters threaded through an introducer. The midline catheter, which is usually 6" to 8" (15 to 20 cm) long, terminates in the axilla. The PICC, which is usually 20" to 24" (51 to 61 cm) long, is advanced into the central venous system and terminates in the superior vena cava. Both require sterile conditions for placement and routine care, and both should be heparinized to maintain patency.

Placement begins with setting up a sterile field. The venipuncture site (which may be the brachial, cephalic, median cephalic, or median basilic vein), is prepped thoroughly. The suggested prep consists of soap, povidone, alcohol, and povidine again. Be sure to allow the patient's skin to dry after each step of the prep, especially the povidone steps. After measuring the appropriate length of catheter needed, the catheter is cut (if necessary) and patency of the catheter is determined by a saline flush before it is inserted.

Venipuncture with a break-away needle or introducer is performed. The stylet of the introducer is removed from the introducer. The catheter is then threaded into the introducer slowly until properly placed. When the catheter is in place and venous access is attained, the stylet is removed and the catheter is aspirated for blood return and flushed to verify patency. RNs should receive training on insertion of the PICC before attempting this procedure because proper use of the equipment is essential. Some PICC and midline catheters enable you to flush during the procedure with the guidewire still in place. This unique feature helps check patency and blood return as the procedure progresses. It also is helpful to be able to keep the guidewire in for better enhancement during X-ray.

The final step is to securely tape the catheter with sterile tape and to apply a pressure dressing for the first 24 hours. This dressing can be changed to a transparent dressing the next day. Placement of the PICC must be verified with an X-ray before use (this is not required for midline catheters).

Complications can arise with these catheters, as with any other type of catheter. Measuring the middle upper arm circumference once daily is a good way to watch for infiltration. The most common complication is occlusion. Thorough flushing and heparinization are essential. Some manufacturers, such as TACY medical, offer a video to purchasers that illustrates placement procedure, catheter dressing instructions, and declotting procedure.

Hickman catheter and Broviac catheter

The Hickman and Broviac catheters are indwelling, long-term CV devices that are surgically inserted through an incision in the deltopectoral groove and advanced into the central venous system and superior vena cava, terminating just before the right atrium. The catheter is tunneled subcutaneously and exits in an area that allows the patient to care for the site and port. The surgeon sutures the catheter in place via a Dacron polyester cuff that adheres to the surrounding tissues; this further secures the catheter and helps prevent entrance of bacteria.

Once the cutdown and exit sites heal, only the external catheter is visible. The patient or nurse can infuse anything from intermittent medications to chemotherapeutic drugs. Blood samples can be obtained and blood can be transfused through the catheter. Patients with such disorders as hemophilia, sickle cell anemia, or cancer and those who receive numerous blood transfusions may benefit from these catheters. Their design decreases anxiety in patients who may require numerous blood withdrawals or infusions over long periods.

The Broviac catheter is identical to the Hickman catheter, except that the Broviac catheter has a smaller inner lumen. Another type, the Hickman-Broviac catheter, combines both units into one catheter. These are excellent catheters for home I.V. therapy because they can be left in place indefinitely, provided no complications develop. The most common complication is occlusion with blood or I.V. solution precipitate, which can occur if the catheter is not properly flushed. Catheter breakage also is a problem. A clamp on the external catheter may be used in case of leakage or breakage. Never use metal clamps directly on the catheter because they may cut the catheter.

Groshong catheter

Another catheter used for long-term CV access, the Groshong catheter consists of thin-walled, translucent silicone with an encapsulated barium sulfate radiopaque strip and a patented two-way slit valve adjacent to a rounded, closed tip. A small Dacron cuff attached to the catheter promotes growth of fibrous tissue, which helps secure the catheter and reduces the potential for infection.

The two-way valve allows easy infusion of fluids and aspiration of blood samples. Under normal central venous pressure conditions (1 to 6 mm Hg), the valve remains closed, reducing the potential for air embolism and flashback of blood through the catheter, making routine clamping of the catheter unnecessary. The valve is designed to remain closed between pressures of − 7 and 80 mm Hg.

The Groshong catheter is flushed with an isotonic fluid (bacteriostatic normal saline solution) once weekly when it is not in use. It also is flushed after withdrawing blood and administering I.V. infusions. Heparinization is not necessary because the two-way valve does not allow blood to enter the catheter. It is recommended that the catheter be flushed, using aseptic technique, with no less than 10 ml of bacteriostatic normal saline solution. After a blood transfusion or withdrawal of blood, *vigorous* irrigation with 20 ml of bacteriostatic normal saline solution is necessary to completely flush the catheter of residual blood, which may inhibit or prevent proper catheter functioning.

The Groshong catheter is available as a single- or triple-lumen catheter. When using the triple-lumen type, be sure to thoroughly flush each lumen with bacteriostatic normal saline solution after using any solution other than plain isotonic solutions.

Implanted ports

The completely implanted port (such as the Infuse-A-Port, Port-A-Cath, and LifePort) provides CV access for blood withdrawal, I.V. solution infusion, blood transfusions, and chemotherapy. The device consists of a self-sealing injection port, reservoir, and a silicone catheter. It may be used to deliver or extract fluids to a selected vessel or body site.

Implanted ports are available in various styles. These devices may require accessing from the top or the side of the device. Side-accessing ports are becoming less common. The ports may come in single- or double-port styles. Familiarity with the exact port placement is essential to avoid accessing the wrong port, which can damage the entire port system.

All implanted ports require two incisions for surgical placement. Two incisions are made in the upper quadrant of the right or left side of the chest: one for port placement (in a pocket and sutured in place); the other for catheter placement (in a cutdown fashion). Both incisions are sutured closed, and the device is completely implanted under the skin.

Because the entire port is implanted and there is no external device to access the port, the septum (or septums) of the port is accessed by feeling for the center of the port and then penetrating the skin and septum with a special needle. *Remember:* Penetrate the septum with a Huber needle only, and heparinize the port regularly when it is in a blood vessel. Also heparinize the port when withdrawing the Huber needle; the heparin that remains in the port and the catheter will help prevent clots.

A common problem with implanted ports is damage caused by improper access. If the Huber needle is not properly placed, the septum can become damaged and leaking can occur. Tissue damage could result from the leaking solution. The catheter must be heparinized; if not done properly, it will become occluded.

Huber needles (noncoring)

These special needles, designed for use in implantable ports, allow for safe and proper penetration of the septum. Because they are non-coring needles, they contribute to the longevity of the device. Ranging from 19G to 24G in size and ½" to 2½" (1.25 to 6.35 cm) in length, the needles are available with 90-degree angle and straight-needle designs.

Some manufacturers offer an infusion set with a Huber needle attached for easy access to the ports (any noncoring needle may be used at any manufacturer's port). Wings for secure taping and attached extension tubing are included to prevent site manipulation. The chance of coring the septum is minimal with an infusion set because it can be well secured. (For more information, see *Noncoring Needles*, page 47.)

Caring for long-term CV devices

Follow the general guidelines below when caring for a long-term CV device.

● On the day of catheter insertion, change the dressing to observe the suture sites and report the amount and type of drainage noted.

Because of subcutaneous manipulation, swelling and serous drainage are expected. It is a good idea to clean the site and redress it, at least twice a day (or as needed).

● Until drainage ceases, use a gauze dressing for absorption purposes.

NONCORING NEEDLES

Unlike a conventional hypodermic needle, a noncoring needle has a deflected point, which slices the port's septum instead of coring it. Noncoring needles come in two types: straight and right-angle.

Generally, expect to use a right-angle needle with a top-entry port, and a straight needle with a side-entry port. When administering an I.V. bolus injection or continuous infusion, you will also need an extension set.

Conventional hypodermic needle

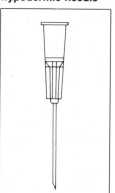

Straight noncoring needle

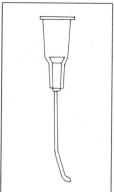

Right-angle noncoring needle

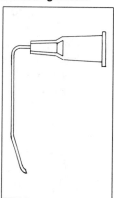

Right-angle noncoring needle with extension set

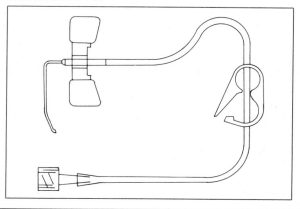

- Once drainage stops, use a transparent dressing. The site should be cleaned and dressed according to policy or according to the physician's orders (refer to the manufacturer's recommendations for optimal use of the dressing).
- Use aseptic technique when changing dressings, and clean the site with a circular motion working from the center outward.
- Remember that patient teaching is essential, especially if the catheter is a long-term indwelling device that will be cared for at home. Encourage the patient to participate in the care and use of the catheter as soon as he or she is physically able.
- Urge the patient with an external catheter, such as the Hickman catheter, to carry a catheter clamp. If the catheter is cut or begins to leak, it will be crucial to clamp it above the leak (between the patient and the leak) to minimize blood loss. Metal clamps should be avoided because they can cut or destroy a catheter. If metal clamps are used in an emergency, a piece of gauze or even a piece of clothing between the clamp and the tubing will protect the tubing from damage.
- With implantable ports, use only Huber needles for venous access. Their design prevents coring of the septum. If the noncoring needle does not have its own extension tubing attached, attaching a T-port between the Huber needle hub and the I.V. tubing greatly reduces pressure on the needle. The device also has an extension that can be clamped during tubing changes to prevent air from entering the port. Heavy tubing attached to the hub of the Huber needle tends to further bend the needle to a 90-degree angle, occluding the infusion. Be sure to tape the needle and tubing securely to prevent circular movement of the needle in the septum. If the Huber needle does not lie flush with the chest, pad it with gauze. This supports the angle and helps prevent further bending.
- With the Groshong CV catheter, be sure to flush the catheter well (vigorously with 10 ml of normal saline solution), especially after infusion of hypertonic solutions.
- Heparinize lumens not used continuously to prevent clotting. Use the following procedure:
  — Prepare equipment and lumen ports (according to hospital procedure).
  — Flush the port with normal saline solution (this determines patency and position and flushes preexisting medication from the I.V. line and cannula). The amount of saline used should be at least two to four times the amount the lumen holds.
  — When flushing I.V. catheters, make it a rule to never use a tuberculin syringe. Flushing should not exceed 25 to 40 psi, or else damage to the catheter could result. The tuberculin syringe would exceed 40 psi and cause too much pressure on the catheter.

—Flush with heparin solution (usual concentration is 100 units of heparin per 1 ml of normal saline solution; however, 10 units is becoming more popular). Be sure to use enough normal saline and heparin solutions (for example, 5 ml) to flush the lumen entirely, from the port to catheter tip.

• If the catheter becomes damaged, an over-the-guidewire procedure is possible to replace the damaged catheter without another needlestick. This procedure should only be done by a trained clinician or a physician. A manufacturer's repair kit should be available.

• If purulent drainage is noted from the insertion site or an infected catheter is suspected, it will be necessary to obtain a culture of the catheter tip. INS recommends the following procedure:

—Withdraw blood from the catheter for culture.

—Clean around the catheter site.

—Do not cover the insertion site as the catheter is removed.

—Remove the catheter in an upward direction to avoid contacting the skin as much as possible.

—Cut the tip end with sterile scissors and save it in a sterile container.

—Withdraw blood from a peripheral site.

Withdrawing blood from the catheter and a peripheral site is recommended to verify sepsis. A semiquantitative sample will identify the organism, then the number of colonies. This will determine if the culture is positive or negative. If the colony count is 14 or less, the culture is negative; 15 or more, the culture is positive.

• If the CV line appears to be obstructed because the solution is not flowing, do not automatically assume that it is clotted. Try moving the patient into various positions, asking the patient to cough, or raising the patient's arms above the head. The obstruction may be caused by the catheter's lying against the vein wall; repositioning and coughing could correct the problem. If the line is clotted, try to aspirate with a syringe at the catheter hub to remove the clot and open the system. If the attempt is unsuccessful, the catheter may require use of urokinase for declotting. For information about this procedure, see the section on "Declotting long-term catheters" below.

• Never infuse any solution other than an isotonic solution before X-ray verification of catheter placement.

• Never try to use any equipment without receiving instruction or without reading the manufacturer's guidelines, especially when penetrating or treating the circulatory system.

• In a code situation, be especially careful when pushing medications through any long-term cannula because too much pressure can puncture or pop the catheter open, resulting in damage, such as infiltration or catheter embolism.

• Review your facility's policies and procedures and the manufacturer's recommendations for long-term indwelling cannulas to ensure safe, optimum patient care.

Catheter occlusion

Catheter occlusion may result from mechanical obstruction, such as kinked tubing, closed clamps, clogged injection caps, clogged I.V. filter, I.V. pump malfunction, or an empty I.V. bag. If these problems are resolved, normal catheter function will return. Other mechanical problesm leading to obstruction of I.V. flow include:

- pinch off syndrome, which occurs when the clavicle presses against the first rib, thus obstructing the catheter.
- lodging of the catheter tip against the vein wall.
- malpositioning of the catheter occurring during insertion or resulting from catheter migration.

Vascular access devices (VADs) may become occluded, regardless of the type of device or placement of the cannula tip. A common problem, fibrin accumulation in or around the catheter, may cause secondary problems if left untreated. These include:

- loss of venous access
- inability to use same site for later venous access
- risk of catheter infection caused by bacterial or fungal colonization.

Examine the I.V. setup for kinked tubing, closed clamps, empty infusion bags, and malfunctioning pumps. Ask the patient to change position to see if catheter position can be changed. Check for tight sutures on external catheters. Finally, a chest X-ray may be helpful to confirm catheter placement and rule out catheter tip migration.

Catheter occlusion also may result from non-thrombotic obstruction. Mineral deposits and lipid-based precipitates may occlude the catheter. A 3-in-1 soution that contains lipids as well as other additives is more likely to cause occlusion than intermittent infusion of lipids alone. Common causes of precipitate formation include:

- incompatible pH of drugs and solutions
- admixture technique
- electrolyte ratios
- I.V. flow rates
- flushing and heparinization procedures.

Non-thrombotic occlusions may be difficult to detect. Methods for catheter clearance (such as the use of hydrochloric acid) do exist, but they are rarely used. Frequently, urokinase is used to rule out thrombus formation, which may lead to a decision to remove and replace the catheter.

Catheter occlusion resulting from thrombus formation can occur rapidly, possibly within 24 hours of insertion. Such occlusion may result in clotted blood or accumulated fibrin in the catheter, platelets or fibrin encasing the catheter surface, a fibrin tail extending from catheter tip, thrombus along the vessel wall that causes endothelial damage, deposits forming within the reservoir of the port, or deposits or fibrin accumulating around the outlet tube of the port.

Declotting long-term catheters

All of the long-term CV devices discussed above are prone to catheter occlusion. If thrombotic occlusion is verified, declotting the device with urokinase is possible. (*Note:* Always obtain a physician's order before attempting to declot a CV catheter.) The following procedure may be used when a small amount of urokinase (1.8 ml) is needed:

- Remove all of the tubing connected to the hub of the catheter.
- Attach a three-way stopcock to the hub of the catheter.
- Place an empty 10-ml syringe at the 90-degree angle of the stopcock.
- Place a 10-ml syringe with urokinase at the other port of the three-way stopcock.
- Turn the stopcock off to the urokinase.
- Aspirate 9 ml of air from the catheter into the empty syringe. (This creates negative pressure in the catheter.)
- While holding the empty syringe at the 9-ml mark, turn off the stopcock to the empty syringe and turn it toward the syringe with urokinase. This will pull in the appropriate amount of the urokinase to fill the space in the catheter created by the negative pressure created upon aspirating the 9 ml of air.
- Allow the urokinase to remain in the catheter for no less than 15 minutes. Then aspirate the urokinase from the catheter.
- If you cannot aspirate blood from the catheter, repeat the procedure; procedure may be performed up to 4 times. After 1 hour, urokinase loses its potency.

Note: Never allow the urokinase to enter the bloodstream. Always aspirate the urokinase from the catheter before flushing.

The procedure using negative pressure works best on soft catheters. Another method, in which urokinase is pulsated into an occluded catheter, is reserved for triple-lumen catheters because they are not as pliable as other long-term catheters. The pulsation method may rupture more pliable long-term catheters.

CONTROLLERS AND PUMPS

Infusion control devices are designed to infuse I.V. solutions and medications with a more consistent, reliable rate than can be delivered without such a device. Electronic devices save nurses time by maintaining control over the rate of the infusion. They also provide a sense of security by detecting air in the tubing or catheter and by detecting whether an I.V. container is empty.

Controllers

A controller device administers I.V. solution with the aid of gravity. Therefore, the I.V. container must be at least 30″ to 36″ above the level of the heart. The controller has an electronic eye that is positioned on the drip chamber to measure the drops of fluid administered. A change in gravity may interrupt the device, and an alarm may sound if resistance in the I.V. line, such as from a clot or infiltration, occurs.

Pumps

Numerous types of pump devices are available and all do exactly what they say—they "pump" solution into a vein. This means that solution is administered under pressure. Some pumps share similar features; however detailed in-service instruction is necessary to ensure proper use. Refer to the manufacturer's manual to determine how your facility's pump works, and follow its recommendations for use and maintenance.

Common types include infusion pumps, volumetric pumps, syringe pumps, multichannel pumps, self-powered pumps, patient-controlled analgesia (PCA) pumps, and implanted pumps.

- *Infusion pumps* are used to control the rate of flow (in drops/minute or milliliters/minute), providing an increased level of safety to the infusion. They reduce the risk of air embolism and circulatory overload.
- *Volumetric pumps* measure the volume being delivered in milliliters (usually milliliters/hour). These pumps may rely on peristaltic movement over the tubing to move the fluid or on a piston cylinder unit (also called cassette) to pull fluid into the cylinder and push it out much like a syringe.
- *Syringe pumps* are used to administer small doses of high-potency drugs and administration of I.V. push medications in a more consistent fashion using a syringe under pressure. They also save valuable nursing time. These pumps may be used to infuse medications given consistently or intermittently.
- *Multichannel pumps* provide the user with one programmable pump that is much like using four pumps. They can be programmed to administer four different medications with flushes in between doses. Administration of medication can be done via an I.V. bag, bottle, or syringe.
- *Self-powered pumps* are used most often in the home setting. It uses the internal pressure that is created once it is filled. They are used for slow, continuous infusion of medications.
- *Patient-controlled analgesia (PCA) pumps* are used for patient administration of analgesics as needed for pain control. The device has a lock-out system that prevents the patient from overdosing.
- *Implanted pumps* are designed for slow, continuous, low-volume, long-term I.V. infusion. These devices are surgically implanted and contain medication chambers that can be filled and refilled by the physician. The infusion of the medication is activated by heat. The device is completely implanted and requires no care between refills.

Electronic infusion pump devices vary in size, cost, and capability and are equipped with an alarm system that indicates complications. The complications may include air in the line, empty container, occlusion, machine malfunction, low battery, and open door.

One important issue about using pumps is integrity of the vein. The delicate vein walls do not handle high pressure over long periods.

This is especially true for elderly patients. Always check your patient's pump for pressure settings. The ability to change the pressure (measured in psi) on the pump may prolong vein integrity. High-pressure settings are acceptable when administering an infusion via a central I.V. line, but low- to medium-pressure settings should be used with peripheral lines. High-pressure settings used on peripheral lines may actually cause infiltration.

Like a controller device, a pump can aid in infiltration detection by sounding an alarm. The pump detects an increase in resistance as pressure builds from the infiltration, thereby sounding the alarm. Although it is true that the pumps can detect an increase in resistance, such as when the tubing kinks or becomes occluded, do not fall into the trap of relying on the pump for detecting infiltration. An I.V. solution administered to a young patient via the pump at a rate of 100 ml/hour will sound the alarm much faster than the same I.V. infusion administered to an elderly patient. The reason is the patient's skin tone. An older person's skin will hold quite a bit more solution than a younger person before the same amount of resistance is detected by the pump.

A pump should be carefully checked for proper pressure settings, especially when elderly patients are involved. Remember that your eyes are still the best detector of infiltration. When using a pump, frequently observe the I.V. site for signs of infiltration, and feel and compare the site to the same area on the other arm. This is *always* the best way to detect I.V. complications of any kind.

I.V. DRESSINGS

Various I.V. dressings and taping techniques may be used to secure the venipuncture device and protect the I.V. site from infection and other complications. Many facilities are now using a semipermeable transparent dressing, which secures the device directly to the patient's skin, eliminating the need for tape and allowing an unobstructed view of the I.V. site. In any case, the I.V. site should remain clean of blood and debris and be covered at all times. Sterile dressings and aseptic technique should always be used. Depending on institutional policy, a small amount of topical antimicrobial or antibiotic ointment may be applied over the I.V. site before the dressing is secured.

Before applying an I.V. dressing, remember to check the patient's skin condition and determine whether the patient is allergic to any substances in the ointment or dressing. If the patient has thin, delicate skin, use minimal tape or consider applying paper tape to avoid tearing the skin when removing the tape for dressing changes.

When choosing a dressing, keep in mind the patient's condition and type of I.V. therapy. Gauze dressings do not keep the catheter site as secure as transparent dressings do; also, they tend to cover the insertion site and inhibit routine observation. Transparent dressings leave the insertion site visible and provide added security to the stabilization of the cannula. Transparent dressings also allow evaporation of moisture from the skin. Some transparent dressings, such as the OpSite IV3000, not only allow evaporation from the skin, but also pull moisture away from the skin to the surface of the dressing. This is especially important for central I.V. line dressings; clean, dry central I.V. line sites are very important to decrease growth of bacteria and colonization.

Securing the I.V. dressing involves more than just randomly applying of a few pieces of tape (for more information about specific taping methods, see *Taping Techniques,* pages 55 and 56). Routinely observe the I.V. site every time you enter the patient's room, and change the dressing every 24 to 48 hours, or as needed.

I.V. infusion site maintenance

Keep in mind the following general guidelines when maintaining the I.V. dressing site:

- Apply antimicrobial ointment according to institutional policy.
- Keep ointment application to a minimum; too much causes the tape to loosen.
- Completely cover the insertion site with a sterile. semipermeable dressing.
- Keep the site and the dressing clean and dry.
- Avoid securing the dressing too tightly to ensure patient comfort.
- Apply ½"-wide tape chevron-style, approximately 1" above the catheter hub to prevent manipulation of the I.V. line.
- Use paper tape when the patient's skin requires delicate treatment.
- Use a minimum amount of tape.
- Use T ports as appropriate to prevent cannula manipulation during tubing change.
- Apply a clear dressing for easy observation of the infusion site.
- *Remember:* Securing tape to tape on I.V. dressings greatly increases the security device and allows for safe, easy tape removal. Never place gauze under the cannula hub without first covering it with tape. Tape positioned over the top of the gauze and hub will capture the hub between the gauze and tape, making tape removal for site care very difficult.

The following recommendations are made by INS for securing the I.V. line and caring for the insertion site:

- Apply a topical ointment (if used) to the I.V. site at the time of insertion. The use of an antimicrobial ointment (such as povidone-iodine) is preferred and widely accepted. However, some researchers suggest that the use of polyantibiotic ointment may be effective at the skin-catheter junction and that antiseptic and/or antimicrobial ointments (such as povidone-iodine) have only marginal benefits.
- A sterile dressing (preferably a transparent, semipermeable membrane adhesive dressing) should be applied over all I.V. sites to cover the catheter entrance site.

TAPING TECHNIQUES

Use one of the five taping methods described here to secure your patient's I.V. site.

Chevron method
1. Cover the venipuncture site with an adhesive strip or a 2″ × 2″ sterile gauze pad. Then cut a long strip of ½″ (1.25 cm) tape. Place it, sticky side up, under the needle, parallel to the short strip of tape.
2. Cross ends of tape over the needle so that tape sticks to the patient's skin.
3. Apply a piece of 1″ (2.5 cm) tape across the two wings of the chevron. Loop the tubing and secure it with another piece of 1″ tape. On the tape, write the date and time of insertion, the type of needle gauge, and your initials.

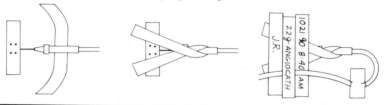

U method
1. Cover the venipuncture site with an adhesive strip or a 2″ × 2″ sterile gauze pad. Then cut a strip of ½″ tape. With the sticky side up, place it under the tubing.
2. Bring each side of the tape up, folding it over the wings of the needle, as shown here. Press it down, parallel to the tubing.
3. Now apply tape as you would with the chevron method. On the tape, write the date and the time of insertion, the needle or catheter gauge, and your initials.

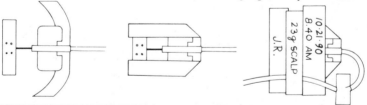

Two-Tape method
1. Cover the venipuncture site with an adhesive strip or a 2″ × 2″ sterile gauze pad. Then place a 2″ (5 cm) strip of ½″ tape, sticky side up, under the needle.
2. Fold tape ends over, and affix them to the patient's skin in a U shape, as shown.
3. Place a second strip of ½″ tape, sticky side down, over the needle hub. On the tape, write the date and time of insertion, the type of needle or catheter gauge, and your initials. With this method, you can remove the upper strip of tape to inspect the insertion site while the lower strip anchors the needle.

(continued)

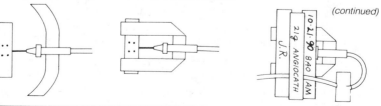

TAPING TECHNIQUES *(continued)*

H method
1. Cover the venipuncture site with an adhesive strip or a 2″ × 2″ gauze pad. Then cut three strips of 1″ tape.
2. Place one strip of tape over each wing, keeping the tape parallel to the needle.
3. Now place the other strip of tape perpendicular to the first two. Put it either directly on top of the wings or just below the wings, directly on top of the tubing. On the last piece of tape, write the date and time of insertion, the needle or catheter gauge, and your initials.

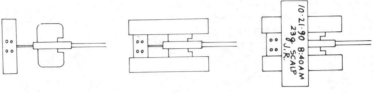

Transparent semipermeable method
1. Remove the dressing from the package and, using aseptic technique, remove the protective seal. Avoid touching the sterile surface.
2. Place the dressing directly over the insertion site and the hub, as shown. Do not cover the tubing. Also, avoid stretching the dressing; doing so may cause itching.
3. Tuck the dressing around and under the catheter hub to make the site occlusive to microorganisms. To remove the dressing, grasp one corner, then lift and stretch.

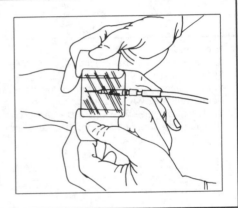

● Change I.V. dressings every 24 to 48 hours or immediately if the dressing becomes soiled, wet, or loose. (*Note:* The newer transparent dressings may remain in place for longer periods. Check the manufacturer's packaging for recommendations.)

The Centers for Disease Control and INS have recommended that hospitals develop standard policies and procedures to ensure optimal delivery of I.V. care. Patient allergies and skin conditions may warrant the use of nonstandard equipment. Aseptic technique and accepted practices can only benefit the patient.

Because of the vast array of I.V. equipment on the market, gaining familiarity with all types is difficult. However, being aware that there are alternatives should help. Your patient may benefit greatly from a certain T port, catheter plug, extension tubing, or long-term indwelling catheter. As a nurse, you may be able to recommend a piece of equipment to the physician or your patient. Knowing that the equipment exists may be as important as knowing how to use it.

4 SETTING UP AN I.V. INFUSION

Because each institution uses different I.V. equipment, describing all of the various types of setups is impossible. Therefore, this chapter will address the safe, efficient way to to set up a standard gravity-flow I.V. line. Regardless of the type of I.V. setup, however, always keep the setup as simple as possible without compromising care. Also, keep in mind that the patient pays for each piece of equipment added, so economize whenever possible, considering the patient's needs.

The first step in setting up an I.V. infusion is to read the physician's orders carefully to ensure that you fully comprehend the written order and any special instructions. Be especially alert to the possiblility of allergies. If any part of the order seems unclear or you know that the patient has an allergy that may preclude the use of a particular solution, notify the physician at once.

After verifying the proper I.V. solution to be administered, determine which I.V. setup to use. Selection of the appropriate equipment can mean the difference between a troublesome I.V. line and a trouble-free one. Before selecting the tubing, consider the following:

● Which solution is to be infused?

This is the most important consideration when deciding which type of tubing to use. The type of tubing must be compatible with the solution; in some cases, special tubing may be required. For example, the chemical compositions of nitroglycerin and Taxol require non-polyvinyl chloride tubing to prevent these solutions from adhering to the tubing wall or impeding infusion rates.

● What is the rate of infusion?

The infusion rate is another important consideration. *Remember: Enough fluid must move through the I.V. catheter to prevent gravity from pulling blood back into it.* Decreased movement allows blood and solution to become stagnant in the catheter, which may result in a clogged I.V. line. This is especially important when the I.V. rate is less than 50 ml/hour. Almost any tubing will deliver more than 50 ml/hour adequately. If less than 50 ml/hour is needed, microdrip tubing should be used.

● What type of I.V. monitoring device, if any, is to be used?

Some pumps and controllers require specially manufactured I.V. tubing designed specifically for the device. Be sure to check the device for any special requirements.

● What is the patient's activity level?

The tubing length should be appropriate for the patient's activity level, so consider whether the patient is on bed rest or allowed bathroom privileges. For instance, if the patient is ambulatory, shorter tubing may be necessary to prevent the patient from accidentally tripping over the tubing. Tubing that is too long may be cumbersome and may impede gravity flow.

● Where will the I.V. site be located?

Site location may require the use of extenders, such as extension tubings or T ports, to minimize manipulation of the I.V. site and prevent complications.

CALCULATING INFUSION RATES

I.V. rates can be calculated in many different ways. Regardless of the method used to calculate the rate, it is important to know the drop factor of the tubing, the amount of fluid to be infused, and the amount of time over which the fluid is to be infused.

The longer, more detailed classroom method of calculting I.V. rates is as follows:

$$\frac{\text{Amount of fluid} \times \text{Drop factor}}{\text{Time of infusion (in minutes)}} = \text{Drops per minute}$$

The drop factor is noted on the manufacturer's package. It indicates the number of drops the set must deliver according to drop size to obtain one milliliter of solution. It is measured in drops/ml. The formula shown above is long, and calculating it may take precious time. Consider the following, more practical method when on the nursing unit:

$$\frac{60 \text{ (minutes)}}{\text{Drop factor}}$$

The drop factor divided into 60 minutes will give a number to be divided into the ml/hour ordered. This "magic" number is constant, depending on the tubing used. I.V. tubing is manufactured in four drop factors: the minidrip (microdrip) drop factor is 60 drops/ml; the maxidrip (macrodrip) drop factors are 10, 20, and 15 drops/ml. (Note that *drop* is commonly abbreviated *gtt.*)

MINIDRIP	MAGIC NUMBER
60 gtt/ml	1 (60 divided by 60)

MAXIDRIP	MAGIC NUMBER
10 gtt/ml	6 (60 divided by 10)
20 gtt/ml	3 (60 divided by 20)
15 gtt/ml	4 (60 divided by 15)

As you can see, the magic number remains constant. So, whenever a 60-drop factor set is used, the ml/hour (noted on the I.V. label) is divided by 1. Whenever a 10-drop factor set is used, the ml/hour is divided by 6. Whenever a 20-drop factor set is used, the ml/hour is divided by 3. And, whenever a 15-drop factor set is used, the ml/hour is divided by 4.

The ml/hour rate should always appear on the I.V. label; calculating the drops/minute will be easy. Remember that the infusion time in hours divided into the amount to be infused gives the ml/hour. Try the following examples:

1. An I.V. infusion of 1,000 ml of dextrose 5% in water (D_5W) is to run at 125 ml/hour. The tubing used delivers 20 drops/ml. What is the rate in gtt/minute?

$$60 \div 20 = 3$$
$$125 \div 3 = 42 \text{ gtt/minute}$$

Every time a 20-drop tubing is used, divide the ml/hour by 3.

2. An I.V. infusion of dextrose 5% in one-half normal saline (0.45% sodium chloride) solution is to run at 175 ml/hour. The tubing used delivers 10 drops/ml. What is the rate in gtt/minute?

$$60 \div 10 = 6$$
$$175 \div 6 = 29 \text{ gtt/minute}$$

Every time a 10-drop tubing is used, divide the ml/hour by 6.
This method gives a standard number,

$$60 \div \text{drop factor} = \text{"magic number"}$$

which is to be divided into ml/hour. It is an easier method to use at the bedside because the "magic" number is a constant number. Use the longer formula in a classroom situation to show the calculations, and then check it with the easy method.

Note: To use the bedside method, you need to divide the ml/hour rate by the "magic" number specific to the drop fctor being used. Don't mistakenly divide the ml/hour rate by the drop factor itself.

The number of drops per milliliter (gtt/ml) listed in *Comparing Infusion Rates,* page 60, represent the highest numbers possible used to deliver the desired rate. By comparing the rates in the chart, you will see that microdrip tubing (60 gtt/ml) maintains catheter patency better than tubing with a larger drop factor, but it may not be the easiest to count for accurate infusion rate. Keep in mind that rates ordered at 50 to 75 ml/hour can be maintained with tubing of any drop factor. However, when rates below 50 ml/hour are ordered, minidrip tubing is best. Conversely, for rates greater than 75 ml/hour, maxidrip tubing is best. This will guarantee using the best tubing to maintain patency and make the rate countable. The formula to remember is: minidrip < 50 to 75 ml/hour > maxidrip.

A handheld I.V. calculator (I.V. Checkset) provides an accurate and reliable method for determining I.V. flow rates and checking prescription compliance for I.V. medication dosages. It instantly calculates and

COMPARING INFUSION RATES				
The chart below identifies the appropriate infusion rate for I.V. infusions using I.V. tubings with different drop factors. Minutes are abbreviated as "min" in this chart.				
	Ordered rate			
Drop factor	**20 ml/hour**	**50 ml/hour**	**100 ml/hour**	**125 ml/hour**
60 gtt/min	20 gtt/min	50 gtt/min	100 gtt/min	125 gtt/min
20 gtt/min	7 gtt/min	17 gtt/min	34 gtt/min	42 gtt/min
15 gtt/min	5 gtt/min	13 gtt/min	25 gtt/min	32 gtt/min
10 gtt/min	4 gtt/min	9 gtt/min	17 gtt/min	21 gtt/min

displays I.V. infusion rates as drip rates (drops/minute), flow rates (milliliters/hour), or infusion rates (hours and minutes) when the "drip count" button is pressed. It also calculates the remaining infusion time at the current flow rate setting and will automatically determine flow rate settings for dosage compliance using familiar formulas prebuilt into the device. This type of device can help reduce errors in calculation, thus promoting accurate, reliable, and safe I.V. infusions.

ASSEMBLING EQUIPMENT: SPECIAL CONSIDERATIONS
Careful planning is necessary when setting up an I.V. infusion. After considering the type of infusion solution, the prescribed rate, the monitoring device to use, the patient's activity level, the length of the tubing, and any necessary add-on devices, the next step is to gather and assemble the equipment. After setting up the system, attach it to the hub of the cannula before entering the patient's room. Having the system ready for venipuncture will spare the patient from watching and waiting anxiously for a needlestick to be performed.

When a patient is receiving medications that need controlled, slower rates or careful titration, microdrip tubing is necessary. Aminophylline, lidocaine, and dopamine infusions are examples requiring accurate delivery rates. Electronic infusion devices also should be used with these infusions, but always check whether special tubing is needed. Some machines deliver up to a specific number of gtt/minute; other devices are set according to gtt/ml. A problem arises when a rate is ordered as 75 ml/hour and the machine can only be set up to 69 ml/hour. In this case, microdrip tubing would not be adequate.

You will save time and avoid wasting equipment if you are familiar with your facility's infusion monitoring devices and their specific tubing requirements before choosing the I.V. tubing. (Note that electronic infusion devices are not covered in detail in this book. Be sure to consult your education department and/or the manufacturer's representatives for information on the machines used in your facility.)

If a patient is restless or frequently is out of bed, make sure the length of tubing is not uncomfortable or inconvenient for the patient's needs. For example, longer tubing may be needed to prevent a restless patient from accidentally pulling out the I.V. cannula, whereas shorter tubing may prevent an ambulatory patient from tripping on the I.V. line. Also, keep in mind that tubing that is too long can impede the gravitational flow of the I.V. solution.

If a patient is switched from an intermittent to a continuous I.V. infusion, do not use a needle to pierce the I.V. lock cap and connect the continuous infusion. Instead, remove the catheter cap and connect the tubing directly to the catheter hub or T-set hub.

Finally, T ports, add-on filters, and extension sets may be beneficial to use with your I.V. setup. They can provide extra tubing length, extra injection ports, and easy accessibility for tubing changes without disturbing or soiling the dressing. However, they also present new areas for leakage and separation of the I.V. line and increase the risk of contamination from handling. Using luer-lock connections and taping junctions can help decrease the incidence of separation. If ports are taped, the ends of the tape should be tabbed for easy removal.

SETTING UP THE INFUSION

The best advice for any nurse who is setting up an I.V. line is to be prepared. Have the appropriate equipment ready before proceeding with the venipuncture. Also, remember to tape the ports to prevent separation and to tape the roller clamp. The basic steps for setting up an I.V. infusion are outlined in *How to Set Up a Gravity Flow I.V. Infusion*, pages 62 to 64.

Hanging the I.V. solution on an I.V. pole will maintain the fluid at an adequate height for the proper rate of infusion. The fluid level should be 30" to 36" above the level of the heart to maintain a consistent gravity infusion rate. A change in height may alter the flow rate.

Infusion pumps and controllers are highly recommended, especially for patients receiving medications that require titration. They help prevent fluid overload and the inadvertent bolus administration of medications. The infusion device will sound an alarm when the bag is empty, to alert the nurse of the need for more solution or to indicate an occlusion or air in the line. Check the machine immediately when the alarm sounds.

Be sure to mention to the patient and visitors that the I.V. flow rate is set by the roller clamp (or machine) and is best left untouched. A safe practice, especially with pediatric patients, is to put tape around the roller clamp to prevent anyone from moving the controlling device.

HOW TO SET UP A GRAVITY FLOW I.V. INFUSION

The following steps should be taken when setting up a gravity flow I.V. infusion. When handling equipment, keep in mind that gloves generally are not necessary when attaching tubing to the I.V. solution. However, when connecting the tubing to the patient, gloves must be worn to reduce the risk of blood exposure.

Procedure step	Rationale
1. Inform the patient of the procedure.	**1.** Understanding the procedure helps to alleviate anxiety and encourages the patient to verbalize questions, fears, or concerns.
2. Gather the necessary equipment, such as an I.V. pole, solution, appropriate tubing, add-on devices (extension tubing), and control devices (flow regulators, pumps), before approaching the patient.	**2.** Equipment preparation saves time and minimizes patient anxiety.
3. Check the solution to ensure that it was prepared as ordered and is free of contaminates, cloudiness, color changes, and particulate matter.	**3.** Such safety precautions are necessary to ensure that you are delivering the right solution to the appropriate patient. Careful observation of the solution is necessary to prevent contamination.
4. Wash your hands.	**4.** Always use aseptic technique when setting up the I.V. infusion to prevent contamination and transmission of infection.
5. Slide the roller clamp up to a level close to the drip chamber.	**5.** This allows better visualization of the drops and easy accessibility to the flow control device. If the roller clamp is low on the tubing, it can become lodged under the patient or in the sheets.
6. Close the clamp.	**6.** This prevents inadvertent airflow and excessive fluid flow into the patient. It also affords the user more control over the speed of solution when the solution begins running through the tubing.
7. Remove the protective cover from the spike.	**7.** Removing the protective cover maintains sterility of the devices until they are ready for use. If the I.V. solution in a bottle contains a latex diaphragm, be sure to remove the diaphragm. If you cannot hear the breaking of a vacuum-seal, consider the solution to be contaminated.
8. Spike the bag or bottle without touching the sterile port or spike. If spiking a bag, hang it from the I.V. pole first. If spiking a bottle, invert it and rest it on a firm, stationary surface before pressing the spike into the largest port (the spike port).	**8.** Spiking the bag or bottle without touching it maintains the sterility of the system.

HOW TO SET UP A GRAVITY FLOW I.V. INFUSION *(continued)*

Procedure step	Rationale
9. Gently squeeze the drip chamber until the chamber is one-third full.	**9.** Squeezing forces fluid from the I.V. container into the drip chamber. Underfilling the chamber can result in air pockets; overfilling the chamber will make it difficult to visualize the drops.
10. Open the clamp, and prime the tubing.	**10.** Proper priming is necessary to ensure proper functioning and to expel air from the tubing, which can lead to an embolism.
11. Invert and tap all filters and ports as the fluid approaches.	**11.** This action releases trapped air from the infusion line. Note that some filters must not be tapped while filling. Read and follow manufacturer's instructions to be sure which filters can be tapped.
12. Avoid touching any unprotected connections with your hands or other objects. Also, avoid touching the tubing's protective cap when priming the tubing.	**12.** All male and female connections must be protected from contamination. Keep in mind that the tubing's protective cap will be replaced later and therefore must remain free from contamination.
13. Clamp the tubing.	**13.** Clamping stops the flow of fluid through the tubing. Some tubings have caps that vent air, so removing the protective clamp may not be necessary.
14. Replace the protective cap at the end of the tubing.	**14.** Replacing the cap prevents the end of the tubing from becoming contaminated. Note that, if the cap vents air, replacing the cap will not stop the fluid flow.
15. Loop the tubing over the I.V. pole.	**15.** This keeps the tubing from touching the floor, which may lead to contamination.
16. Label the tubing, indicating the date and time it was started or the date it is to be chnaged, according to institutional protocol.	**16.** This ensures that appropriate tubing changes are made.
17. Once placement of the catheter is complete, remove the protective cap at the distal end of the tubing and connect the tubing to the hub of the I.V. access device. Without touching the end of the tubing where the cap was, be sure that the connection between the hub and the tubing is secure.	**17.** This ensures a sterile, closed system.

(continued)

HOW TO SET UP A GRAVITY FLOW I.V. INFUSION   *(continued)*

Procedure step	Rationale
18. Secure the catheter and the tubing before removing your hand.	**18.** Be sure the weight of the tubing will not dislodge the I.V. cannula by securing the device before letting go of the tubing. This ensures a secure, closed system and helps prevent complications.
19. Initiate the flow of solution.	**19.** The solution should be started as soon as possible to prevent stasis of blood that may clog the catheter and to verify proper placement of the catheter before dressing the site.
20. If using an infusion device, set the desired rate before performing venipuncture. If no device is being used, adjust the clamp until the correct number of drops/minute is being administered.	**20.** Setting the rate prior to venipuncture makes it easier to use one hand to start the infusion. Make a habit of setting the rate as part of the infusion setup so that, when the tubing is connected to the cannula, pushing start on the infusion device is all that is needed. This way, you can focus your attention on securing the cannula.

5

SELECTING AN I.V. SITE

Intravenous therapy involves accessing the venous system (veins) rather than the arterial system (arteries). Doing so successfully requires a thorough knowledge of the anatomy and physiology of the vascular system. This chapter will review this system and discuss factors to consider when selecting an I.V. site.

REVIEW OF THE VASCULAR SYSTEM

Successful venipuncture becomes easier if the nurse is knowledgeable about systemic circulation, the aorta, arteries, arterioles, capillaries, venules, and veins. Of major concern in I.V. therapy is the veins, which are divided into three classes:
- superficial (also called cutaneous) veins
- deep veins
- venous sinuses.

The superficial, or cutaneous, veins are used for venipuncture. They are found in the superficial fascia, just under the skin. They sometimes join with the deep veins, especially in the legs. The deep veins are not recommended for venipuncture because of the high potential for thrombus formation, which may lead to pulmonary embolus.

Arteries and veins share certain characteristics: both are composed of three layers of tissue called tunica.
- Tunica adventitia, the outer layer of the vessel, contains connective tissue that surrounds and supports the vessels. This layer is thicker in the arteries than in the veins.
- Tunica media, the middle layer, contains muscle, elastic tissue, and nerve fibers. This layer maintains the vessel tone and is responsible for constriction and dilation.
- Tunica intima, the innermost layer of the vessel, consists of a layer of smooth, flat cells that is only one cell thick, allowing blood cells to flow without interruption. Valves exist in the semilunar folds of this layer, primarily in veins; they prevent the backflow of blood and keep the blood flowing toward the heart. This layer can be easily destroyed by catheter insertion and manipulation, predisposing the patient to phlebitis and thrombosis. (For more information, see *Anatomy of Arteries and Veins,* page 66.)

Arteries are under greater systemic pressure than veins and do not contain valves. Arteries also pulsate and are anatomically deeper, being protected from injury by tissue and muscle. Arteries can be accessed with the same catheters used for venous access. Arterial access usually is performed by physicians; however, in some hospitals, specially trained nurses can access arteries.

ANATOMY OF ARTERIES AND VEINS

The illustrations below show the three layers of an artery and a vein. Understanding the anatomy of the veins can help you to locate appropriate venipuncture sites and to perform venipunctures with minimal patient discomfort.

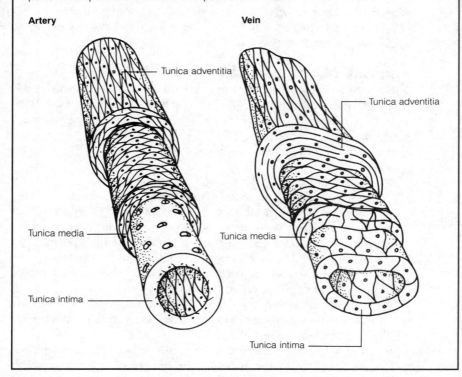

Artery

Vein

Veins respond to the pressure of the circulatory system, but not directly. For example, a patient who has a high blood pressure reading or a pregnant patient with increased blood volume may have more venous distention. The middle layer is not strong or stiff, so the veins collapse or distend with changes in blood pressure. Conversely, the heart exerts a constant pressure on arteries, which prevent their collapse, but they spasm frequently.

In many cases, veins require the application of a tourniquet above the venipuncture site to remain distended and accessible for venipuncture. A tourniquet exerts pressure on the vein, trapping blood and impeding venous flow. Valves located in the vein's inner layer act as a one-way door, allowing the blood to flow only toward the heart. Consequently, the vein becomes engorged with blood between the valves and tourniquet, thus stabilizing the vein and making the vein more visually prominent.

Insertion of a catheter into a vessel will cause some trauma to the vessel, regardless of how well the technique is performed. Soft, well-tapered, thin-walled catheters and gentle technique will greatly reduce the trauma. Traumatic venipuncture, which damages the endothelial layer (tunica intima), predisposes the vessel to phlebitis and thrombosis.

Catheter peelback and movement in the vessel also cause trauma to the inner vessel wall. Remember, the innermost layer is only one cell layer thick and can be easily stripped away. The vessel will become irritated, causing an influx and aggregation of fibrin and platelets. Phlebitis and thrombosis can develop, causing pain and scarring.

Another important issue is skin integrity. The skin is made up of two layers: the epidermis and the dermis. The epidermis, the outer covering, protects the dermis. The thickness of the epidermis differs, depending on its location and the person's age. The palms of the hands and the soles of the feet are covered with a thicker epidermal layer than the forearms. With aging, the epidermis becomes thinner, decreasing support of the veins used for venipuncture.

The underlayer, or dermis, is vascular and contains thousands of nerve fibers. The concentration of nerve fibers varies with different areas, resulting in diverse sensitivities to touch, pressure, temperature, and pain. Therefore, inserting a needle in one area may be more painful than in another.

Also important is the superficial fascia, or subcutaneous connective tissue, which lies below the dermis. This layer, which contains superficial veins and varies in thickness, is susceptible to infection (cellulitis) because of the looseness of the tissue. Asepsis is especially important because bacteria easily spread in this loose tissue.

PERIPHERAL VENOUS SITE SELECTION

If you are inexperienced at performing a venipuncture, be sure to thoroughly review the anatomy of the peripheral veins first (for more information, see *Peripheral Venipuncture Sites,* pages 68 and 69). Practice applying a tourniquet on healthy classmates, family members, and friends; note closely how their veins look, feel, and react to touch. Note any palpable or visual nodules; these may be valves, which may prevent proper insertion and threading of the catheter, so remember to always avoid inserting a catheter just below them.

Keep in mind that venipuncture is possible even without a tourniquet. This is especially significant when performing a venipunture on an elderly patient, who may have delicate veins that will not withstand the extra pressure. Remember that areas from the fingertips to the shoulders can be used for peripheral venipuncture sites.

It is important to choose a venipuncture site carefully. Generally, starting in the hand or wrist area is recommended, so that the veins

(Text continues on page 70.)

PERIPHERAL VENIPUNCTURE SITES

When selecting a venipuncture site, keep in mind that the superficial veins in the dorsum of the hand and the forearm offer the most choices. The dorsum of the hand contains many small, superficial veins that can be easily dilated to accommodate a needle or catheter (left). The basilic, cephalic, and median antebrachial veins of the forearm are generally long and straight and have a fairly large diameter (right); they are especially useful for venipunctures involving large-bore needles and long catheters. If the veins in the hand or forearm are too impractical to use, consider using the veins in the feet or legs. For infants under age 6 months, the scalp veins commonly are used.

For a comparison of the advantages and disadvantages of venipunctures involving the veins in the hand and forearm, see the chart below.

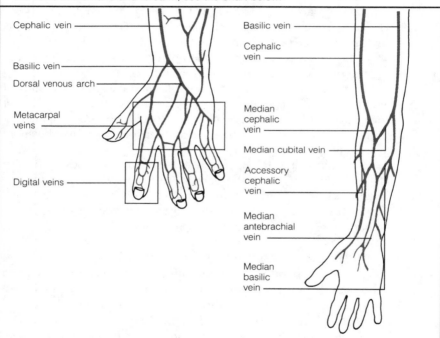

Site	Advantages	Disadvantages
Digital veins Run along lateral and dorsal portions of fingers	• May be used for short-term therapy. • May be used when no other means are available.	• Fingers must be splinted with a tongue blade, decreasing ability to use hand. • Uncomfortable for patient. • Infiltration occurs easily. • Can't be used if veins in dorsum of hand already used.

(continued)

PERIPHERAL VENIPUNCTURE SITES *(continued)*

Site	Advantages	Disadvantages
Metacarpal veins On dorsum of hand; formed by union of digital veins between knuckles	• Easily accessible. • Lie flat on back of hand. • In adult or large child, bones of hand act as splint.	• Wrist movement is decreased unless a short catheter is used. • Insertion is more painful because there are more nerve endings in the hands. • Site becomes phlebitic more easily.
Accessory cephalic vein Runs along radial bone as a continuation of metacarpal veins of thumb	• Large vein excellent for venipuncture. • Readily accepts large-gauge needles. • Doesn't impair mobility. • Doesn't require an armboard in an older child or adult.	• Sometimes difficult to position catheter flush with skin. • Usually uncomfortable. Venipuncture device is inserted at bend of wrist, so movement causes discomfort.
Cephalic vein Runs along radial side of forearm and upper arm	• Large vein excellent for venipuncture. • Readily accepts large-gauge needles. • Doesn't impair mobility.	• Proximity to elbow may decrease joint movement. • Vein tends to roll during insertion.
Median antebrachial vein Arises from palm and runs along ulnar side of forearm	• Vein holds winged needles well. • A last resort when no other means are available.	• Many nerve endings in area may cause painful venipuncture or infiltration damage. • Infiltration occurs easily in this area because of joint movement.
Basilic vein Runs along ulnar side of forearm and upper arm	• Will take a large-gauge needle easily. • Straight strong vein suitable for large-gauge venipuncture devices.	• Uncomfortable position for patient during insertion. • Penetration of dermal layer of skin where nerve endings are located causes pain. • Vein tends to roll during insertion.
Antecubital veins Located in antecubital fossa (median cephalic, located on radial side; median basilic, on ulnar side; median cubital rises in front of elbow joint)	• Large veins facilitate drawing of blood. • Often visible or palpable in children when other veins won't dilate. • May be used in an emergency or as a last resort.	• Difficult to splint elbow area with armboard. • Median cephalic vein crosses in front of brachial artery. • Veins may be small and scarred if blood has been drawn frequently from this site.

up the arm remain accessible for future sites. (If you begin in the forearm and the site becomes red and sore, using sites below the forearm for subsequent venipunctures could cause more pain and redness because the I.V. solution may flow through the previously irritated vein.) However, be sure to consider your patient's lifestyle and needs when choosing a vein. An active, self-sufficient patient needs the use of the hands and the ability to bend his or her arms. For such a patient, avoiding the hands and antecubital areas is suggested.

Special considerations

Always assess the patient's activity level before employing hand veins for I.V. infusion. A patient who is manually active may dislodge the catheter. Keeping the dressing dry also may be difficult because of hand washing. The metacarpal veins may not be the best location, depending on the patient's level of activity and cooperation.

- Although the fingers may be used for venipunctures, these sites can be uncomfortable. Also, because of the smallness of the veins, they are not recommended for solutions or drugs being infused at high rates. It is important to splint these sites well for proper solution flow and adequate catheter life.
- Securing an I.V. line on the flat surface of the hand is generally easy; however, if the tip of the catheter lies near the wrist, bending the joint can obstruct the vein, decreasing the flow of solution. Using an armboard can prevent irritation at the catheter tip and ensure that the I.V. flow is not impeded.
- Inserting an I.V. line in the wrist area is not recommended for an agitated patient because of the possible need for wrist restraints. If restraints are necessary, apply them directly to an armboard; then apply the armboard to the patient's arm around the I.V. site to avoid positioning the restraint directly on the site. Secure the patient's arm with double-back tape to protect the I.V. site from trauma and to keep the site visible for routine observations. Remember, taping tightly can cause venous obstruction, so be careful to avoid taping too close to the catheter tip.
- Keep in mind that your choice of an I.V. site for a dehydrated or extremely ill patient may be severely limited; such a patient may have only one available vein, perhaps in a finger. Long-term I.V. therapy may present many problems, and venipuncture may be frustrating and painful for the patient. Choosing the best available vein is essential to decrease the stress involved.
- Avoid using veins that are suspected of being sclerosed or "rolling."
- Avoid using leg veins unless they are specified by a physician or they are necessary for the patient's condition. If lower extremities are used, the Intravenous Nurses Society recommends changing the cannulas as soon as a satisfactory site can be established.

CENTRAL VENOUS SITE SELECTION

The nurse must be thoroughly familiar with the anatomy of the central venous system to peripherally insert a central venous catheter because of the risk of complications. Placement and care of catheters in these veins should be done using strict aseptic technique because of the veins' direct route to the heart.

The vessels involved in the central venous system include the cephalic vein, basilic vein, axillary vein, jugular vein, subclavian vein, innominate vein, and superior vena cava. The pathway of central circulation begins with the cephalic and basilic veins.

The cephalic vein travels up the arm along the outer border of the biceps, terminating in the axillary veins at the upper one-third of the arm. The basilic vein, which has a larger diameter than the cephalic vein, terminates in the axillary vein, but its path is along the inner portion of the upper arm along the biceps.

The axillary vein increases in size as it ascends to a point just below the clavicle. This is where the axillary vein becomes the subclavian vein. A landmark for the beginning of the subclavian vein is the outer border of the first rib.

The subclavian vein is joined by the external jugular vein, which travels from the head along the carotid plexus of the neck. It continues to the inner end of the clavicle, where it joins the internal jugular vein to form the innominate vein. Valves are present until just before the innominate vein.

The innominate vein on the left side is approximately 2½" (6.4 cm) long and has a larger diameter than the one on the right, which is only 1" (2.5 cm) long. The left innominate vein descends slightly and crosses the front of the chest from left to right.

The superior vena cava is formed where the right and left innominate veins meet. It descends vertically down the right side of the sternum, beginning at the first rib, and empties into the right atrium of the heart.

FACTORS TO CONSIDER WHEN CHOOSING A VENIPUNCTURE SITE

When preparing for a venipuncture or caring for an I.V. site, nurses tend to focus mainly on where the catheter enters the skin. However, regardless of where the catheter is placed, keep in mind that the catheter tip itself is equally important because this is where the solution is flowing from. If the tip is occluded, the flow rate will be impeded. So, before insertion, always visualize where the tip will be after the venipuncture to ensure that the catheter will fit in the vein properly.

Also take time to inspect the patient's left and right arms for the most suitable vein. Choosing an I.V. site hastily may cause the patient unnecessary pain and frustration and may result in higher equipment costs.

FACTORS AFFECTING I.V. SITE SELECTION

1. Duration of I.V. therapy

1. For a patient who requires long-term therapy, it is necessary to start as distally as possible. (Avoid fingers if possible.) Alternate arms and veins. Evaluate the patient's veins and the course of therapy, and choose the appropriate type of venous access that will be safe for the duration of therapy.

2. Catheter size

2. Hemodilution is important to prevent vein irritation. According to Intravenous Nurses Society standards, the catheter's gauge should be as small and as short as possible. The appropriate size for most situations is a 20G to 22G catheter. Larger catheters generally are used for large veins, short-term venous access (such as withdrawing blood), surgery, and trauma when the administration of large volumes of fluid is the goal.

3. Type of solution

3. High-pH, low-pH, and hypertonic solutions can be irritating. Hemodilution will be important. Selecting a large vein is necessary to handle the solution and ensure hemodilution.

4. Condition of the vein

4. Soft, straight veins are the best choice. Move your finger down the vein and observe how it refills. Sluggish fill may indicate a vein that is prone to collapse. Avoid veins that are bruised, red, swollen, or located near a previously infected area. Always restart an I.V. infusion above another site, not below it. Laboratory punctures, unsuccessful I.V. insertion attempts, or previously discontinued I.V. sites may render a vein unsuitable for I.V. infusion. Previously used veins can leak and cause infiltrations if the solution is allowed to go through them again. Avoid used veins, especially if the solution is a vesicant (one that causes tissue damage).

5. Patient's level of consciousness

5. Patients in restraints may have fewer areas where the I.V. line can be inserted. The wrists and probably the lower forearm should be avoided to accomodate the restraint. If these areas have the best available veins, the restraint can be wrapped around an armboard and then secured to the I.V. site. Do not wrap the restraint around the I.V. site itself. This could lead to pulling out of the I.V. line and increases the risk of infection and mechanical phlebitis.

6. Patient activity (observe how the patient functions)

6. If a patient is ambulatory and using crutches or a walker, avoid the wrist and hands because the patient needs these to function. The veins of the forearms and upper arms are best because they are naturally splinted and free of joints.

7. Patient's age

7. Infants do not have as many accessible sites as older children and adults. Children under age 4 still have a high percentage of baby fat. Veins in the hands, feet, and antecubital region may be the only accessible ones. Veins in elderly patients are usually fragile and should be approached gently. Extremely fragile veins can be penetrated without a tourniquet; however, caution is needed because excessive pressure may rupture the vein wall when punctured. Rupture of the vessel can lead to "flooding" of blood in the area, thus making venous access impossible.

FACTORS AFFECTING I.V. SITE SELECTION *(continued)*	
8. Hand dominance	**8.** Although the dominant hand usually has the most available veins, avoid using it whenever possible to prevent limiting an active patient and to avoid overactivity of the arm receiving the I.V. infusion.
9. Existing disease or chemotherapy	**9.** Patients with vascular disease or dehydration may have limited venous access. Patients on chemotherapy may have poor venous access and poor vein texture.
10. Dependent edema	**10.** Occasionally, venous distention actually makes venipuncture easier. However, venipuncture will be difficult if serious edema is present in surrounding tissue. With prominent veins, such as a radial vein or veins of the hand or inner forearm, the fluid can be manually pressed out of the area, making the vein visible. If the patient is restrained, look under the restraint for a vein. Pressure from the restraint causes fluid to disperse and makes the vein visible.

Remember that the best I.V. site is one that:
● tolerates the I.V. rate without difficulty
● delivers the prescribed medications adequately
● is comfortable to the patient
● adequately tolerates the gauge and length of catheter needed for the patient and procedure
● does not compromise the patient's activities of daily living.

Special procedures, tests, and surgery also can affect I.V. site selection. The I.V. site may have to be in the right or left arm for a specific procedure, or a specific gauge catheter may be necessary, such as during surgery. Most facilities have policies and procedures regarding special requirements for I.V. therapy. Knowing the patient's history and needs will also be a factor in selecting an I.V. site. (For more information about other factors to consider, see *Factors Affecting I.V. Site Selection.*)

6

PERFORMING THE PROCEDURES

This chapter focuses on the various procedures connected with starting and stopping I.V. infusions, administering local anesthetics, and troubleshooting problems.

STARTING AN I.V. LINE

Most nurses learn how to start an I.V. line simply by doing it, since hands-on experience is the best teacher. Even though the common goal is to access a vein (in the direction of blood flow—toward the heart), nurses typically develop their own insertion techniques. Regardless of the technique used, it is important to always follow hospital procedure and maintain asepsis when performing a venipuncture.

Keep in mind that your approach toward the patient and the procedure will be the first step in your success. Maintain a calm, confident attitude, and the patient will trust in your skills. If you are attempting a venipuncture for the first time, refrain from letting the patient know this. And never tell a patient that you want to "practice" on his or her veins; such a statement is likely to cause anxiety and vasoconstriction in the patient.

Catheter insertion is the part of the procedure most nurses fear. In many cases, nurse can feel and even see the vein, but may be unable to insert the catheter into the vein. Unfortunately, the only way to overcome this fear is by trial and error. Check to see whether your facility can supply an artificial arm for practice sessions before attempting venipuncture on a patient. This will enable you to develop a sense of coordination so that patients will not recognize you as a beginner.

Develop a feel for inserting each of the various catheter types. Over-the-needle catheters seem to provide safer I.V. therapy for a larger group of patients, especially children, because a more flexible catheter remains in the body. Also, the absence of a needle makes nurses and patients less likely to worry about complications.

ADMINISTERING A LOCAL ANESTHETIC

Some controversy surrounds the use of local anesthestics, such as lidocaine, for I.V. line insertion. Although the final decision about using an anesthetic probably should rest with the individual patient, you may need to educate the patient first. Keep in mind the following points:

- A lidocaine wheal tends to obliterate the vein, making it more difficult to see and feel.
- Using lidocaine involves two needle sticks instead of one.
- Lidocaine is usually an extra cost to the patient.

- A lidocaine injection often is very painful. Some patients think it is more painful than the venipuncture itself.
- Lidocaine is associated with certain complications. Some patients are allergic to it.
- Improper placement of lidocaine can lead to cardiac complications and death.
- Lidocaine should only be considered necessary for large-gauge catheter insertion.

Use of eutectic mixture of local anesthetics (EMLA) cream is another option. A topical anesthetic used in various procedures requiring local anesthesia, EMLA cream is placed on the preferred area and covered with a transparent dressing. The cream must stay in contact with the skin for at least 45 minutes for the desired effect for venipuncture; therefore, it should not be used for procedures that cannot be delayed for 45 minutes. Complications associated with the use of EMLA cream are minimal. Although local allergic reactions have been reported, the cream is considered very safe to use. It is especially helpful when placing an I.V. line in a child and when inserting a large-gauge peripherally inserted central catheter (PICC) or midline catheter.

CATHETER INSERTION

The general procedure for inserting a catheter and initiating I.V. therapy is outlined in *Initiating I.V. Therapy,* pages 76 and 77. Some helpful hints and suggestions for successful catheter insertion are listed below.

- If your facility's budget allows, try using various types of catheters to become acquainted with their different designs (see Chapter 3, I.V. Equipment, for a discussion of the various types). Typically, most nurses become proficient with using one type or a specific design. This can pose problems when the design of the "preferred" catheter predisposes the patient to complications. For example, the Intima catheter (Becton-Dickenson) is a helpful design for use in most situations, especially those involving elderly patients with delicate veins and skin. However, the Intima is not available in gauges larger than 18G, so it may not be appropriate for trauma victims or some surgical patients.
- Study the arms of friends who have prominent veins. This will provide real-life practice in vein selection. Feel them. Run your finger down the vein briskly and notice the vein refill behind your finger. This is a sign of healthy venous refill.
- Take the time to feel for the best vein possible. Keep in mind that the visible veins are not always the best. Palpate for a more significant vein, feeling for a slight "bounce," while pressing your finger across the patient's arm. A more bouncy feeling will indicate the presence of a vein. This method is best because the "bouncy" feeling can be felt even while wearing gloves.

(Text continues on page 78.)

INITIATING I.V. THERAPY

The following general procedure may be used to initiate I.V. therapy.

Inform the patient of the procedure. This helps to alleviate patient anxiety.

Assemble equipment.
This prevents interruption of the procedure if everything is at hand.
Equipment includes:
- catheter
- dressing materials
  - tape (type of tape depends on patient's skin condition)
  - transparent dressing or sterile gauze
  - bactericidal ointment (optional)
  - alcohol or povidone-iodine solution
  - I.V. pole
  - I.V. solution
  - primed and assembled I.V. tubing
- scissors (optional)
- tourniquet
- gloves.

Wash hands.
Hand washing is crucial in preventing the spread of disease.

Apply a tourniquet.
A tourniquet helps to distend the vein. Be sure a radial pulse is present; an absent pulse indicates that the tourniquet is too tight and is obstructing arterial flow.

Select the I.V. site.
See Chapter 5, Selecting an I.V. Site, for specific instructions.

Prepare the site. Be sure to clip the hair in the area rather than shave it.
Proper site preparation minimizes the risk of infection. Shaving can result in microabrasions and increased risk of infection. Less hair also allows better visualization of the vein and facilitates taping.

Prepare the skin. Swab the area with an antiseptic solution, using a circular motion (from inside out) with plenty of friction. Scrub on a disinfectant, such as tincture of iodine, and

leave it on for at least 30 seconds before inserting the catheter.[1]
Proper skin cleansing minimizes the risk of infection. Tincture of iodine (1% to 2% iodine in 70% alcohol) is inexpensive, well tolerated, and probably the most effective disinfectant.

Don gloves.[2]
Make it a habit to wear gloves during I.V. insertion; they prevent cross-contamination from contact with blood.

Anesthetize the area by injecting lidocaine directly over the projected location of venipuncture or by applying eutectic mixture of local anesthetics (EMLA) cream. (Note that this step is optional.)
Use of local anesthesia is controversial. Some believe that the injection of the local anesthetic hurts more than the venipuncture itself, especially when the catheter being used is 20G or smaller.[3] The wheal of anesthetic can obstruct the feel or visibility of the vein.

Penetrate the skin. Hold the catheter as recommended by the manufacturer. Remember that you will need to be able to visualize the flashback, so hold the catheter accordingly. In one steady motion, insert the catheter through the skin with the bevel up. Stop, think, and relax a second. Now, approach the vein.
This allows space to maneuver the catheter appropriately and provides an opportunity to become familiar with skin turgor.

Penetrate the vein.
A slower approach allows for more control and less vein trauma. Once blood return appears, stop.
If using a scalp-vein needle, lift up on the vein very slightly and advance gently into the vein.

INITIATING I.V. THERAPY (continued)

If using an over-the-needle catheter, two techniques are acceptable: Slide the catheter off the stylet, into the vein. Or, slightly advance the stylet to be sure the catheter tip is also in the vein; then remove the stylet and advance the catheter into the vein. *Note:* Do not forget to dispose of the stylet properly in an impervious container.

Both methods prevent puncture of the vein on the opposite side when removing the stylet. *Never* reinsert the stylet into the catheter because of the possibility of slicing the catheter.

Release the tourniquet.
Once blood return is obtained and the catheter is in place, remove the tourniquet to allow venous blood flow to return to normal.

Connect I.V. tubing to the hub of the catheter.
With the catheter in proper position, the I.V. solution can be connected, maintaining a closed system.

Slowly turn on the I.V. infusion and watch for signs of infiltration.
Allowing the solution to run into the catheter rapidly can cause the vein to spasm and clamp down on the catheter (this often occurs in small children). The I.V. solution may not run immediately, but once the spasm ceases, it will begin to run. If infiltration occurs, discontinue and restart the I.V. line at another location. *Never* use an irritant or vesicant solution to test a newly inserted I.V. line.

Set the I.V. solution to run slowly until a dressing is applied.
The dressing should be occlusive (site covered and tubing anchored to prevent kinks). Tape should not be wrapped around the entire extremity (this causes venous constriction, which can result in infiltration).

Set the I.V. at the ordered rate.
Setting the rate ensures accurate fluid delivery. If this was done earlier, this is a good time to double-check.

Inform the patient about possible complications, and explain the need to report any redness, swelling, or pain. Also, tell the patient to have the I.V. site reinforced if the tape loosens.
Early detection allows for prompt treatment of complications. If the dressing loosens, site contamination is likely.

Remove gloves and wash hands. Always avoid contact with the patient's blood.
This prevents cross-contamination between patients.

Label the catheter. On a piece of tape, write the type, gauge, length, insertion date, and your initials. Apply the tape close to the dressing for easy identification.
Labeling ensures good communication among health care team members.

Chart the procedure. Be sure to include the catheter gauge, added equipment (such as extension tubing), dressing applied, site preparation (include clipping of hair), rate of I.V. infusion, and how the procedure was tolerated. Also, include the fact that the patient was informed of signs and symptoms of complications.
Accurate documentation also ensures good communication.

---

[1]Maki, D.G. "Infections Due to Infusion Therapy," in *Hospital Infections*, 2nd ed. Edited by Vennett, J.V., and Brachman, P.S. Boston: Little, Brown, and Co., 1985.

[2]The Centers for Disease Control recommends that gloves be worn whenever there is a *possibility* of blood exposure.

[3]If time allows, use of EMLA cream, another type of local anesthetic, is much less painful. Only problem with using this anesthetic cream is it must stay in contact with the skin for 30 to 45 minutes before insertion is performed.

- After puncturing the skin, try various approaches for penetrating the vein. Some nurses are more successful by inserting the catheter either bevel-up or bevel-down and by approaching the vein from either the top or the side. The bevel-up approach is recommended as most stylets are designed for bevel-up approaches. Approaching bevel-up and to the side of the vein provides you with a bit more control over the direction of the catheter.
- When attempting to penetrate the skin, be sure to hold the skin taut. This will cause less trauma and pain for the patient. Before insertion, measure the catheter against the vein, and be sure the tip will clear joints and nodules to help ease threading.
- When veins tend to roll or move away, pull down on them slightly below the site of entry. Tension on the vein makes the wall easier to penetrate.
- Do not spend too much time probing. Gently feel for the tip of the catheter. Feeling the tip in relation to the vein should give you an idea of whether the catheter is above, below, to the right, or to the left of the vein. If you cannot stabilize the vein for penetration, or if the vein disappears, remove the catheter and attempt venipuncture in another vein.

Inserting an over-the-needle catheter

Various techniques may be used when inserting an I.V. catheter. Some nurses prefer to stick the patient, obtain a blood return, and push the catheter into the vein while pulling the stylet out. Others may prefer to place the entire catheter into the vein before pulling the stylet out. When inserting an over-the-needle catheter, the "hooded technique" is most often recommended.

To perform the hooded technique, follow these steps:

1. After choosing the appropriate vein for the type of therapy ordered, pierce the skin.

2. Enter the vein at an angle of about 60 degrees, and obtain a blood return.

3. Change the angle of approach by dropping the angle of the catheter to less than 30 degrees. Always line up the catheter with the vein to make sure that the catheter tip will remain inside the vein and not exit vein on one side.

4. Lift up slightly and advance the catheter ¼" (6 mm). This step is very important. *The presence of a blood return indicates that the bevel of the stylet is in the vein, but the catheter may not be.* Catheters sit back on the stylet, and they are tapered in size to the stylet. The hole made by the stylet may not be large enough for the catheter to enter through, especially if the stylet is removed once the blood return is obtained. So advancing the catheter ¼" will ensure that the catheter is also in the vein.

5. "Hood" the stylet. Pull back slightly on the stylet to hide the tip inside the catheter. This prevents the possibility of puncturing the posterior vein wall.

6. Advance the catheter along with the stylet up to the hub. The stylet will act as a guidewire. This is important to ensure that the catheter fits through the hole; it also adds stiffness to the softer catheter materials.

7. Remove the stylet, and add I.V. tubing or a PRN male adapter.

When inserting an over-the-needle catheter, keep in mind the following points:

- Always look closely at the catheter before inserting it. Examine it for plastic "burrs" or obvious manufacturing errors. Notice the small distance between the tip of the stylet and the tip of the catheter.
- After insertion, stop once flashback has begun. Lift up slightly on the vein and insert the catheter a little more to ensure that the tip is in the vein and not just the stylet. Lifting up on the vein helps keep the tip of the stylet in the vein and prevents puncturing the other side of the vein. Slight advancement before removing the stylet ensures that the catheter tip is in the vein. Another method involves inserting the catheter by sliding it off the stylet while holding the stylet's position and maintaining flashback. When using this technique, *never remove the stylet until the catheter is well into the vein.*
- Never reinsert the stylet into the catheter once it has been removed. This can cause piercing or slicing of the catheter, creating a catheter embolus.
- Never insert a needle into a patient more than once. The device becomes contaminated upon insertion into the skin. Attempting to reuse that needle constitutes poor technique.

TROUBLESHOOTING PROBLEMS

Sometimes problems can occur with I.V. catheter insertion. Some common problems and solutions are discussed below.

Problem #1: Blood return stopped. "I went through the vein."

While inserting the catheter, a small blood return was obtained, but it stopped. Can it be fixed? Yes, sometimes — by pulling the stylet back until the catheter can be seen and then slowly pulling the catheter back. When blood enters the catheter, quickly and gently advance the catheter before the vein has a chance to advance. Remember, once the stylet is pulled back, do not reinsert it into the catheter; it might perforate the catheter wall.

Problem #2: Difficulty threading the catheter. "When I push the catheter into the skin, it seems as though I am pushing the vein."

When this happens, the stylet is in the vein and blood return is visible. However, the catheter diameter, which is larger than the stylet, is outside the vein; as the catheter is advanced and the stylet is pulled back, the catheter can push the vein and not enter it. It is possible that the vein is moving as you push the catheter into the skin. Be sure to pull the skin taut below the site of insertion. This will help to minimize vein movement. This is when the "hooding technique" is effective. Once you obtain a good blood return, be sure to advance the catheter ¼″, then pull the stylet back into the catheter. Lift upward on the stylet as the catheter is advanced the rest of the way into the vein.

Problem #3: Difficulty threading the catheter. "I get so excited when I see blood, I forget what to do next and the vein blows."

Other commonly heard statements include: "I know I was in but it would not thread," "The vein blew," or "I don't know what happened, I had a good flashback." All of these statements are indications that you may have overfilled the veins or there was an interruption in the forward movement of the catheter while attempting venipuncture. An overdistended vein may "burst" when punctured; the vein can shrink away after it has "burst," pulling away from the bevel and leaving the bevel out of position to advance the catheter, thereby stopping the blood return. The tip of the bevel also can perforate the skin. Don't overfill the veins. You must continue with a forward motion when a blood return is obtained, or the blood will leak out and the vein will deflate. Continue forward movement and lift gently upward while sliding the catheter along the vein.

Problem #4: Difficulty threading the catheter. "I had a blood return, but I could not feed the catheter in."

It is obvious that the catheter sits back on the stylet and that the catheter is of larger diameter than the stylet. The stylet is used only for puncturing the vein. The catheter must be inside the vein before the stylet is pulled back into the catheter or completely removed. If the stylet is removed too soon, the catheter has no opening to enter the vein, but the blood has a way to exit the vein. This is why the vein "blows." Once blood return is obtained, advance the catheter slightly, then hold the stylet very still while sliding the catheter off the stylet into the vein. Then completely remove the stylet.

Inserting a scalp-vein needle

A scalp-vein needle (SVN), or butterfly needle, is inserted using the same basic technique as an over-the-needle catheter, except that it requires a more delicate approach because a needle is being advanced into the vein. Avoiding the other side of the vein is very important, and hooding is not possible. If the vein is large and straight, this technique is simple. However, if the vein is small and curves slightly, or if it is not visible, the SVN may be difficult to insert without infiltration.

All nurses develop confidence and technique with exposure to various procedures, including insertion of an SVN. Be sure to follow standard procedure and maintain aseptic technique. Keep in mind the points below when inserting an SVN:

- Apply pressure just above the SVN tip or pinch the extension tubing to prevent blood from spilling when the tubing is attached.
- After inserting the I.V. line, secure it to the patient's skin. A secure dressing is an important step in protecting the I.V. site from bacteria; it also protects the vein from mechanical phlebitis and skin trauma. Securing the hub is the first and most important part of the dressing. Without a secure hub, the catheter can eventually work its way out of the vein. (See Chapter 3, I.V. Equipment, for suggestions on securing the catheter hub.)

Applying a dressing

Every nurse develops a dressing design for stabilizing various catheters. The goal is to completely cover the insertion site and prevent catheter manipulation, which can cause mechanical phlebitis. The type of dressing, cooperation of the patient, and tolerance of the vein are other important factors.

The dressing should be applied with tape that does not irritate the patient's skin. Remember that excessive taping does not guarantee security and may be uncomfortable for the patient. Strategically placed tape, however, will provide a secure I.V. site. Experiment with various catheter styles, and keep in mind that the tape is applied to secure the line. Having the limb in a natural position while securing the site prevents later pulling and pinching of the tape.

Be sure to indicate on the dressing and in the chart what type and what gauge catheter was used, the date and time of insertion, and your initials. This is the best way to ensure that the site is rotated every 48 hours, according to Intravenous Nurses Society standards. Also, document how the patient tolerated the procedure and the appearance of the site when the procedure was completed.

DISCONTINUING PERIPHERAL I.V. LINES

Intravenous catheters are removed for various reasons. Some common reasons are included below:

- The physician's order indicates that I.V. therapy is no longer needed.
- The catheter has been in the same position for over 48 hours. Routine I.V. site rotation is required, and other veins are available for venipuncture.
- The I.V. site is red, tender, painful, or swollen, or the catheter is occluded.
- The catheter was inserted during an emergency without proper aseptic technique.

Regardless of the reason for removal, the procedure is the same for all types of catheters (for more information, see *Discontinuing a Peripheral I.V. Line,* page 82). The goal is to completely remove the device from the vein without causing trauma to the vein or surrounding tissues. Always be sure to examine the length of the catheter and the condition of the tip to ensure that an intact catheter has been removed. Document these observations in the patient's chart, detailing the entire procedure and describing the condition of the I.V. site.

DISCONTINUING A PERIPHERAL I.V. LINE

Assemble equipment.
Organization prevents interruption of procedure, and helps to minimize patient anxiety.
  Have the following items available:
- gauze
- tape
- gloves
- antimicrobial ointment (optional).

Inform the patient of the procedure.
This alleviates patient anxiety and encourages verbalization.

Wash hands.
Hand washing for at least 10 seconds with friction before contact with a patient reduces the possibility of cross-contamination between patients.

Turn off the solution.
This prevents the possibility of fluid leaking into the tissue upon withdrawal of the catheter.

Don gloves.
This prevents cross-contamination from contact with blood from a potentially infectious person.

Remove the dressing (pull tape toward the I.V. catheter).
This technique helps prevent accidental, uncontrolled dislodging of the catheter.

Inspect the site, assessing for signs of infection. Culture the site and catheter tip if drainage is noted.
Inspection identifies possible complications early.

Hold sterile gauze over the insertion site, and quickly slide the catheter straight out of the skin. Do not apply pressure until the catheter is out of the skin.
This prevents vein or skin tearing and bruising of the site.

Apply pressure to the I.V. site with sterile gauze instead of alcohol.
Pressure promotes clotting. Alcohol irritates the wound and inhibits clotting.

Note the length and condition of the catheter.
Rule out emboli by ascertaining that the catheter was removed intact.

Do not apply adhesive bandages.
Adhesive bandages do not exert enough pressure to stop bleeding and can irritate the skin.

Inspect the site again. Assess for redness, swelling, and drainage. Treat and report accordingly. Apply a warm compress to the site if the patient complains of tenderness.
Inspection allows you to detect complications early. A warm compress can be soothing.

Apply antimicrobial ointment.
The ointment will help prevent microorganisms from entering the bloodstream. This step is optional.

Apply a sterile 2″ × 2″ gauze bandage, and exert pressure until oozing stops.
Pressure prevents development of ecchymosis and hematoma at the site.

Chart the procedure. For continuity of care and communication among staff members, be sure to include the reason for removal, date, time, condition of the catheter and site, and the amount of fluid absorbed. Also include how the patient tolerated the procedure.
This ensures good communication among staff members.

When removing an I.V. catheter, keep in mind the following points:
- Keep the catheter parallel with the skin upon removal. Do not apply pressure to the skin until the catheter is completely out.
- Apply firm pressure quickly once the catheter is out, and *avoid rubbing the insertion site.*
- Observe the site for complications before and after catheter removal.
- Inspect the device to ensure that no pieces were broken off.
- Do not use adhesive strip bandages as pressure dressings. They are ineffective at maintaining pressure.

Removing pumps and controllers

Be especially alert when discontinuing an I.V. line if the patient has a pump or controller. In March 1994, the Food and Drug Administration (FDA) issued a public health advisory about reports of injuries and deaths from uncontrolled, rapid infusions of medications or fluids with the use of I.V. pumps and controllers. In some cases, the I.V. tubing and bag were removed before the clamp was closed, resulting in a rapid, uncontrolled flow. To prevent this, do the following:
- Close the clamp on the administration set before opening the infusion pump door or when shutting off the pump or controller.
- Place a warning label prominently on the infusion pump to alert users to close the administration set clamp before opening the infusion pump door.
- Use infusion pumps and controllers with anti-gravity mechanisms.
- Use sets that incorporate limited volume reservoir chambers for continuous administration of potentially toxic medications that come in large-volume bags.
- Limit the concentration of medication in the I.V. solution.
- Make sure that all pumps and controllers are regularly inspected and maintained.

Removing intermittent venous access devices

Intermittent venous access devices, such as heparin locks, are treated like any other peripheral catheter. Be sure to flush a heparin lock with normal saline solution (0.9% sodium chloride) when the device is to be removed immediately after administering a medication. This will prevent any irritating medication that may be left in the device from leaking into the surrounding tissue. Even the smallest amount of some medications can cause tissue damage if infiltrated. (*Note:* Heparinization after the last medication infusion is not necessary if the device is to be removed.)

Another type of lock that is not flushed with heparin is commonly used. It remains patent under the principle that flushing with normal saline solution using a positive-pressure flush will prevent the backflow of blood into the catheter. It is thought that the positive-pressure flushing technique, not the heparin (which is very short-acting), is what keeps the catheter patent.

Positive-pressure flushes are done by pushing normal saline solution through a catheter and pulling out while still pushing. If you stop pushing and then pull out, negative pressure is created in the catheter and blood is pulled into the catheter, resulting in a clot. When performed properly, positive-pressure flushing will cause some normal saline solution to be squirted onto the patient's arm when the needle or syringe is removed.

DISCONTINUING CENTRAL VENOUS LINES
The discontinuation of a central line should be done only by nurses specially trained to perform this procedure because it requires the removal of sutures that anchor the catheter. (*Note:* This does not include long-term indwelling catheters, which require surgical removal.)

The reasons for discontinuing a central venous catheter are similar to those for a peripheral line, except for the following:
● A central line may stay in a vein much longer than 72 hours. The patient must be evaluated daily for complications.
● Central lines should be discontinued and a peripheral line started as soon as medically possible.
● Central lines inserted during an emergency should be observed closely for infection because they have a great risk of becoming septic.

For more information, see *Discontinuing a Central I.V. Line,* page 85.

HANDLING COMPLICATIONS
Complications may arise even after a peripheral or central I.V. line is discontinued. Instruct the patient to observe for signs and symptoms of complications. Some complications are described below.
● Even as late as 24 hours after an I.V. line is discontinued, the site may become red and sore. The irritated vein may benefit from a warm compress.
● Ecchymosis may develop after a catheter is removed because of improper or limited application of pressure to the I.V. site.
● The patient is still at risk for thrombosis after an I.V. line is discontinued. Report to the physician any chest, shoulder, or neck pain. Swelling of the catheterized arm and neck vein distention also are serious complications.
● A vein that appears healthy upon removal of the catheter may become hard and ropelike. If the patient voices concern about this, explain that a vein develops scar tissue from the trauma of cannulation and may remain in this condition for a long time. Reassure the patient that circulation is not impaired by the scarring. However, explain that future venipuncture in this area should be avoided and that proximal insertion to this area should be used.

DISCONTINUING A CENTRAL I.V. LINE

Inform the patient about the procedure.
Patient understanding alleviates anxiety and encourages patient to breathe normally.

Wash your hands.
Washing hands for at least 10 seconds with friction will help prevent the spread of infection.

Assemble the equipment.
Equipment needed includes:
● suture removal set
● sterile 2″ x 2″ gauze pad
● one pair of sterile gloves
● one pair of clean (nonsterile) gloves
● container for catheter tip in case culture is necessary
● dressing materials.
   Organization promotes efficiency and prevents disruption of the procedure.

Don clean gloves.
Gloves are necessary whenever there is a possibility of exposure to blood or body fluids.

Loosen and remove tape toward the catheter.
This prevents pulling and accidental dislodging of catheter.

Apply sterile gloves.
This prevents contamination and possible infection.

Examine the insertion site. Observe for drainage. If noted, collect a blood sample from the catheter and a peripheral sample from the catheter tip for culturing.
Careful inspection helps detect complications early. Culturing will identify the cause of infection.

Snip and remove sutures. Then slowly, carefully withdraw the catheter by pulling it straight out, with the patient holding his breath.
Pulling straight out prevents tearing of the skin and vein. Holding the breath will help prevent air embolus.

Apply pressure for 1 minute with sterile 2″ × 2″ gauze pad. (Femoral veins need pressure for 5 minutes.)
Sufficient pressure is necessary for venous occlusion to begin.

Inspect the catheter tip for damage, and evaluate the length of the catheter. Save the tip for culture if drainage is noted at I.V. site.
This assesses the site for purulent drainage and the catheter for possible embolus.

Observe the site for signs and symptoms of complications. Report any redness, swelling, or drainage to the physician immediately.
This will ensure prompt medical attention.

Apply an antimicrobial ointment, and cover the site with a pressure dressing.
The ointment helps occlude the skin opening, which could lead to an air embolus; it also prevents microorganisms from entering the bloodstream.

Document the procedure. Document the date, time, condition of the site and catheter, and that a dressing was applied. Also, indicate whether the physician was notified if redness, swelling, or drainage had been noted. Chart how the patient tolerated the procedure and the amount of I.V. solution absorbed.
Accurate, thorough documentation promotes continuity of care and good communication among staff members.

Remove all pressure dressings in about 1 hour, and examine the site. Reapply pressure only if necessary.
This ensures that venous occlusion has occurred and has been maintained.

Redress the site without applying pressure.
A clean, dry dressing protects the site from microorganisms.

7
COMPLICATIONS

Good nursing care begins with recognizing, diagnosing, and promptly treating problems. Any invasive procedure carries the risk of complications. With I.V. therapy, the patient can have an adverse reaction to the solution administered, the medications infused, and even to the catheter and venipuncture itself. The complications may be local or systemic, or they may begin locally and become systemic (for example, infection at the site may progress to septicemia).

Nurses must be able to anticipate and prevent problems, recognize existing ones, and initiate appropriate treatment. The first step is to determine whether a problem exists by checking the patient's arm. Is there swelling, redness, or pain at the I.V. site? If so, discontinue the I.V. line immediately. Failure to discontinue the line after making such an assessment could constitute negligence.

Other problems may require further investigation. For instance, if an I.V. line is sluggish, determine its patency by checking for a blood return. A blood return can be obtained in one of three ways:
- by applying a tourniquet 4" to 6" (10 to 15 cm) above the I.V. site and lowering the I.V. bag below the level of the heart
- by aspirating solution from below the clamped I.V. line
- by pinching and releasing the tubing.

A patient with small, delicate veins or low blood pressure may not show a blood return even though the line may be functioning perfectly. Very small catheters may be the reason why a flashback does not result, so do not remove an I.V. line simply because a blood return cannot be obtained.

When an I.V. line is discontinued because of complications and therapy is still needed, restart the I.V. line and resume the infusion at another site. Prompt attention given to a problematic I.V. line will preserve the vein and the accessibility of surrounding veins for future venipuncture.

When discontinuing an I.V. line, remember to check the catheter to make sure it was removed intact. If even the smallest piece of the catheter is sliced or chipped off and allowed to remain in the bloodstream, the patient will develop manifestations of catheter embolus. These manifestations include local thrombosis, thrombosis with embolism, septicemia, and acute bacterial endocarditis. (See Chapter 6, Performing the Procedures, for more on discontinuing an I.V. line.)

After discontinuing the I.V. line, apply pressure on the site until it stops bleeding. Sometimes, a small pressure dressing may be necessary to prevent any further bleeding or bruising at the site. If a pressure dressing is applied, remove it within an hour and reexamine the site to make sure that proper clotting has occurred. Also, remember to document the reason for discontinuing the I.V. line, the condition of the site, and the treatment given. Also document whether a new I.V. line was started.

When a patient has an I.V. line, closely monitor fluid intake and output. An accurate account of the intake and output is necessary for controlling fluid overload and ensuring adequate hydration.

No matter what the problem is in I.V. therapy, immediate attention will prevent patient discomfort and further complications. Signs and symptoms of local and systemic complications commonly associated with I.V. therapy, along with their recommended treatments, are discussed below (for more information about complications, see *Common Complications of I.V. Therapy,* pages 88 to 93).

LOCAL COMPLICATIONS

Local complications that may occur with I.V. therapy include infiltration, phlebitis, clotting of an I.V. line, venous spasm, hematoma, and damage to nerves, tendons, and ligaments.

Infiltration

One of the most common complications of I.V. therapy is *infiltration,* the entrance of an infused substance into surrounding tissues rather than into a vessel. An I.V. solution that has infiltrated can be very painful to a patient, especially if the solution is irritating or damaging to the tissues. Medications, such as potassium, chemotherapeutic agents, dobutamine, antibiotics, and nitroglycerin, are only a few of the many substances that are irritating.

Infiltration and extravasation (infiltration of vesicant solution) can lead to serious nerve, tendon, ligament, and tissue damage. Some infiltrated solutions may cause fluid to leave cells, thus increasing swelling. Other solutions can cause blistering. Patients experiencing infiltration commonly report the following:
- the I.V. site feels cold
- the tape suddenly feels very tight
- tingling in fingers
- cold, numb hands.

Immediate action should be taken for all infiltrations, especially if a vesicant is involved. Remove the catheter immediately, and restart the catheter in the other limb. Elevate the infiltrated limb. If an irritant was infiltrated, initially apply a cold compress on limb for 20 minutes to prevent a histamine reaction that may cause tissue damage. Then apply warm compresses to make the patient comfortable. Check with your facility about the preferred treatment used to prevent tissue damage from extravasated irritants and vesicants (see Chapter 10, Chemotherapy, for suggested treatment of extravasation).

Document when the infiltration occurred, how the site looks, the discontinuation of the catheter, the treatment provided, and if the

(Text continues on page 93.)

COMMON COMPLICATIONS OF I.V. THERAPY

As with any invasive procedure, I.V. therapy carries the risk of associated complications, which may be local or systemic. This chart lists some common complications along with their causes, signs and symptoms, and measures for treatment and prevention.

Causes	Signs and Symptoms	Treatment	Prevention
INFILTRATION			
• Catheter becomes dislodged.	• I.V. site is swollen (swollen area may be below I.V. site, depending on elasticity of the patient's skin).	• Place tourniquet above running I.V. site, tight enough to shut off venous flow. If I.V. solution continues to drip, it *must* be infiltrated. Discontinue I.V. line and restart it well above the site of infiltration.	• Make certain that I.V. site is secure. An armboard on flexor areas is helpful. Lift the arm and evaluate for dependent swelling.
• Vein wall becomes weak and ruptures, and solution leaks into the tissue.	• Swollen area may be cooler than rest of skin.	• Hold pressure at site of discontinued I.V.	• Be sure that tape is not too tight — it can constrict circulation.
• Fluid leaks around catheter and out of the insertion site into the tissues.	• I.V. solution runs but may be sluggish and eventually cease to run. • I.V. solution is draining from I.V. site.	• Elevate limb to enhance movement of solution. • Using gauze, apply slight pressure to I.V. site. • Decrease pressure setting on I.V. pump.	• Use of catheters that are flat and easily secured will decrease skin and vein tearing. Do not allow excessive movement of the catheter in the skin. • Use low or medium pressure settings on I.V. pumps.
• Opposite side of vein wall is perforated.	• Blood return may or may not be present. • Pain at the site of swelling may or may not be present. • Skin in area of infiltrate may be pale.	• Apply warm compress to increase circulation and ease the pain. • Encourage patient to use the affected limb.	• When performing venipuncture, lifting the tip of the catheter slightly, once blood return is obtained, will keep catheter tip from perforating opposite side of vein wall.

COMMON COMPLICATIONS OF I.V. THERAPY *(continued)*

Causes	Signs and Symptoms	Treatment	Prevention
BACTERIAL PHLEBITIS			
• Catheter is inserted incorrectly. • Poor hand washing is used. • I.V. site was not prepared correctly. • Poor dressing care or lack of dressing exists.	• Vein is sore and red; drainage is usually present. • Vein may feel cordlike. • Fever may be present.	• Discontinue I.V. line and restart it in another vein. • Apply warm compresses (may be comforting). • Notify physician (culture of drainage and antibiotics may be ordered).	• Practice good hand washing for at least 10 seconds with friction. • Maintain aseptic technique. • Observe site routinely. • Provide routine site care along with proper dressing.
MECHANICAL PHLEBITIS			
• Site is not taped securely. • I.V. line is usually in unstable area (wrist or antecubital fossa). • Catheter is allowed to move around or in and out of site.	• I.V. site may be red and sore. • Redness is present along vein.	• Discontinue I.V. line and restart it in another vein. • Apply warm compresses to encourage circulation and help soothe the patient.	• Avoid using joints as I.V. site if possible. • Tape I.V. line securely. • Do not allow movement of the catheter in and out of the skin. • Use armboard to decrease catheter manipulation.
CHEMICAL PHLEBITIS			
• Vein irritated by medication or solution.	• Vein may feel hard. • Patient may complain of painful, burning sensations. • Redness travels in the direction of the vein, but tends to flare out and resemble a burn.	• Discontinue I.V. line and restart it in another vein. Apply warm compresses for patient comfort.	• Use neutralizing agent whenever necessary, on advice of pharmacist and physician. • Use largest vein available for good hemodilution.

(continued)

COMMON COMPLICATIONS OF I.V. THERAPY *(continued)*

Causes	Signs and Symptoms	Treatment	Prevention
CLOTTED I.V. LINES			
• Blood may back up easily if rate is slower than vein pressure. • The keep-vein-open (KVO) rate may not provide enough fluid movement. • Tape placed on or near the tip of the catheter. • Tape is too tight, causing obstruction of the blood flow and stasis of fluid. • If I.V. site in a flexor area, flow may cease with bending of the limb. • Patients lying on the tubing can obstruct the flow. • Allowing I.V. line to run dry. • Empty I.V. container and blood backing up in I.V. tubing.	• Blood visible in the tubing. • I.V. line does not drip, even with position change of the arm or catheter. • I.V. line drips, but seems to be backing up into the piggyback. • Inability to flush cannula. • Note that I.V. site usually appears normal.	• Verify that the line is actually clotted. • Discontinue I.V. line and restart it in another site. • Hang new I.V. solution container, clear I.V. tubing of air and blood (may need to change tubing), and flush catheter with normal saline (0.9% sodium chloride) solution.	• Use an intermittent access device for patients with KVO rates. • Use I.V. pump, I.V. controller, or ENERGIZER. • Use microdrip tubing for rates < 50 ml/hour. • Prevent tape or restraints from obstructing I.V. flow; apply restraints to armboards; then secure armboards to the limb by taping around the I.V. site. • Use armboards in flexor areas to prevent bending and obstruction of flow. • Change tubing immediately if blood appears and cannot be cleared. • Use air-eliminating filters to prevent clogging when I.V. container runs dry.
VENOUS SPASM			
• Solution is irritating. • Flow rate is too rapid. • Solution is cold or thick. • Initial catheter penetration into a vein.	• Pain traveling up the arm. • Pain distal to the I.V. site.	• Decrease rate temporarily. • Apply a warm compress to the site of pain. • Immediately restart the I.V. line in a larger vein.	• Use a large-bore vein and a small-gauge catheter to promote hemodilution. • Infuse solutions at room temperature.

COMMON COMPLICATIONS OF I.V. THERAPY *(continued)*

Causes	Signs and Symptoms	Treatment	Prevention
HEMATOMA			
• Opposite side of vein wall punctured at time of venipuncture. • Leakage of blood resulting from needle displacement.	• Tenderness occurs at venipuncture site. • Area around site is bruised. • Unable to advance or flush I.V. line.	• Remove venipuncture device. • Apply pressure and warm soaks to affected area. • Recheck for bleeding.	• Choose a vein that can accomodate the size of the device. • Release the tourniquet as soon as successful insertion is achieved.
NERVE, TENDON, OR LIGAMENT DAMAGE			
• Improper venipuncture technique is used, resulting in injury to surrounding nerves, tendons, or ligaments. • Improper splinting or taping with armboard.	• Extreme pain, similar to electrical shock. • Numbness and muscle contraction. • Delayed effects, including paralysis, numbness and deformity.	• Stop procedure.	• Don't repeatedly penetrate tissues with venipuncture device. • Don't apply excessive pressure when taping or encircling the limb with tape. • Pad armboards as well as tape used to secure armboard, if possible.
CIRCULATORY OVERLOAD			
• Too much fluid enters the body. • Delivery of fluid is too rapid for a particular patient. • Inaccurate monitoring of the I.V. line.	• Rise in blood pressure. • Rise in central venous pressure (CVP). • Dilation of veins (visibly engorged neck veins). • Rapid breathing. • Shortness of breath. • Crackles. • Wide variations between fluid intake and output.	• Decrease I.V. to KVO rate. • Elevate head of bed. • Keep patient warm to promote peripheral circulation. • Monitor vital signs. • Administer oxygen, as necessary and ordered. • Notify physician.	• Always monitor intake and output when patient has an I.V. line. • Know patient's cardiovascular history. • Notify physician if wide variation exists between fluid intake and output.

(continued)

COMMON COMPLICATIONS OF I.V. THERAPY *(continued)*

Causes	Signs and Symptoms	Treatment	Prevention
AIR EMBOLISM			
• I.V. line allowed to run dry. • Large gaps of air in tubing (small air bubbles are unlikely to form emboli, but they are a greater risk with central lines). • Connections have become loose. • Connections have come apart.	• Blood pressure drops. • Cyanosis. • Loss of consciousness. • Weak, rapid pulse. • Rise in CVP.	• Notify physician immediately. • Position patient on left side and lower head of bed. If air has entered the heart chamber, this position may keep air on the right side of the heart, where the pulmonary artery can absorb it.	• Check system for leaks. • Give oxygen, as allowed. • Use controlling devices. • Use luer-lock connections. • Clear tubing of air before attaching to I.V. line, and be sure all connections are secure. • Change all solution containers before they become empty.
SYSTEMIC INFECTION			
• Poor aseptic technique was used. • Equipment is contaminated.	• Sudden rise in temperature and pulse. • Chills and shaking. • Blood pressure changes occur.	• Notify physician. • Take cultures of urine, blood, and sputum, as ordered. • Discontinue I.V. line and restart it in other limb. • Culture the discontinued I.V. equipment.	• Maintain aseptic technique. • Keep I.V. site clean and dry at all times. • Keep all equipment clean during use.
SPEED SHOCK			
• Drugs administered too quickly. • Improper administration of bolus infusion (especially additives).	• Flushed face. • Headache. • Feeling of tightness in chest. • Irregular pulse. • Loss of consciousness. • Shock. • Cardiac arrest.	• Discontinue drug infusion. • Begin infusion of dextrose 5% in water at KVO rate. • Notify physician immediately.	• Read package for recommendations about infusions before giving any medications.

COMMON COMPLICATIONS OF I.V. THERAPY *(continued)*			
Causes	Signs and Symptoms	Treatment	Prevention
ALLERGIC REACTIONS			
• Sensitivity to admixtures. • Sensitivity to skin preparation or antibiotic ointment. • Sensitivity to access device.	• Itching. • Rash. • Shortness of breath. • Edema at site. • Generalized body edema. • Increased blood pressure. • Decreased pulse and respirations.	• Slow I.V. infusion to KVO rate. • Notify physician.	• Question patient about allergies. • Check patient's chart and wristband for any noted allergies. • Monitor patient for reactions to iodine preparation and to Teflon or nylon catheters.

swelling at the site appears to be decreasing. Notify the physician that infiltration has occurred and alert physician to the possibility of circulatory problems in the infiltrated limb.

Some common causes of infiltration include:
• insecure taping of catheter, resulting in dislodging of catheter
• patient confusion, resulting in dislodging of catheter
• thin, weak vessel walls (especially in the elderly)
• use of I.V. pumps, resulting in infiltration caused by pressure created by the pump.

Phlebitis
Phlebitis, the inflammation of a vein, is another common complication of I.V. therapy. A vein can become inflamed for many different reasons, even though the resulting signs and symptoms are the same.

The risk of developing phlebitis begins when a catheter is inserted into a vein or the vein is traumatized, causing a disruption of blood flow. Movement of the device in the vein causes endothelial changes. Platelets collect at the injured site and around the catheter tip, and a thrombus begins to form. The aggregated platelets cause a release of histamines, which increase blood flow to the site via vasodilation. Patients feel moderate pain, and slight redness may be observed at the site. The area may also feel warm to the touch.

An increase in capillary permeability allows proteins and fluids to leak into the interstitial space. The thrombus continues to grow, and the immune system causes leukocytes to gather at the inflamed site. When leukocytes are released, pyrogens stimulate the hypothalamus to raise the body temperature. Pyrogens also stimulate the bone marrow to release more leukocytes. Redness and tenderness increase with each step of thrombus formation.

Phlebitis can be painful. The first sign of redness or complaint of tenderness at the I.V. site should be investigated immediately. If the site is covered, remove the tape and dressing and observe the site. Never guess and never procrastinate; take action as soon as possible. Phlebitis will not improve with time; it will continue to progress and cause pain. If infection results, it can prolong hospitalization and lead to increased medical costs.

The Intravenous Nurses Society (INS) recommends the use of a phlebitis scale to report phlebitis. The recommended scale is as follows:

1+ = Pain, erythema, and/or edema at site; no streak; no palpable cord.

2+ = Pain, erythema, and/or edema at site; streak formation; no palpable cord.

3+ = Pain, erythema, and/or edema at site; streak formation; palpable cord.

Phlebitis that is allowed to advance to stage 3+ can cause limited future venous access. A phlebitic vein should not be used again; it may be scarred, and the surrounding area may be red. Restarting an I.V. line near a phlebitic vein makes it difficult for other staff members to determine whether redness is caused by an old site or originates at the present one.

There are three types of phlebitis: bacterial, mechanical, and chemical. Bacterial phlebitis is characterized by purulent drainage, redness, pain, and possible swelling. Culture the drainage, and then remove catheter by pulling it upward, away from the skin. Save catheter in a sterile container for culture. Mechanical phlebitis is characterized by redness starting at the I.V. site and traveling up the vein; it is caused by manipulation of the catheter in the vein. Chemical phlebitis exhibits redness at I.V. site and traveling along vein path, and also may exhibit flare; it resembles a burn. Patient may complain of a burning sensation. It is important to remember that all three types must be observed for and treated as soon as possible. They do not improve unless the catheter is removed; they continue to progress and cause the patient discomfort.

Notify the physician and the infection control nurse of any suspected I.V.-related infection, such as purulent thrombophlebitis or bacteremia. A culture must be taken of the purulent drainage from an inflamed site. If phlebitis is determined to be bacterial in origin, the patient may require antibiotic therapy, resulting in a longer hospital stay. Bacterial phlebitis can cost the patient extra time in the hospital, many doses of antibiotics, and, in rare cases, his life.

Clotted I.V. line

A clotted (or clogged) I.V. line can be particularly annoying for the patient and the nurse, especially because it is the complication that is easiest to prevent. Most clotted lines are ones that have been set at a keep-vein-open (KVO) or to-keep-open (TKO) rate. Keep in mind that the movement of fluid through the catheter or positive pressure is needed to maintain patency. The movement of solution keeps blood from flowing back into the catheter, thereby preventing the formation of blood clots.

Maintaining positive pressure inside the catheter is also a way to prevent blood from backing up into the catheter and forming an occlusion. The procedure for flushing with positive pressure is discussed in Chapter 6, Performing the Procedures, under the subhead "Removing intermittent venous access devices."

The first sign of a clotted I.V. line is the cessation of I.V. fluid flow. If the I.V. solution is being administered with a mechanical infusion device, the machine will sound an alarm to warn of the obstruction. Because visible signs are not usually present at the I.V. site, the site may appear normal and healthy.

If the solution has stopped flowing completely and some sort of obstruction is obvious, first check for kinks in the tubing or roller clamps. Apply a pair of clean (nonsterile) gloves and try to aspirate the clot. With a syringe close to the site, withdraw a little solution or blood from the line, thereby attempting to dislodge and remove a possible clot. If blood is obtained, the line probably is not clotted. Do not aspirate over and over, attempting to remove a clot because this procedure can cause trauma to the vein walls, and may cause phlebitis.

Another way of testing patency is to check the line for resistance. Clamp the tubing; use a syringe containing 1 to 2 ml normal saline solution (0.9% sodium chloride) via a port and gently, *without force,* try to inject the solution through the line. If the patient complains of sharp pain, the clot may have been attached to the vein wall. As it was dislodged, trauma occurred in the tunica intima; this may predispose the patient to phlebitis. If you encounter pressure or resistance, *do not force* the solution into the line. Resistance may indicate a clot at the catheter tip. Forcing could push a clot into the bloodstream, thereby causing pain, vein irritation, and, possibly, an embolus.

Runaway I.V. lines and empty piggybacks infusing into intermittent venous access devices are the biggest culprit. It is very important to continuously monitor the flow of the I.V. solution and discontinue empty solution containers immediately upon emptying. If nothing is moving through the catheter and positive pressure has not been maintained in the catheter, the line will become occluded.

I.V. pumps infuse I.V. solution using pressure measured in pounds per square inch (psi). Pumps have the ability to maintain an I.V. line even when only set at 1 ml/hour. They may divide the 1 ml/hour into increments that maintain positive pressure and movement into the catheter. However, because blood is more viscous, it will back up into the I.V. solution if the limb is lower than the level of the heart. This practice is not recommended for ambulatory patients. The ENERGIZER, a non-gravity saline flushing device, can be connected to I.V. locks and can maintain a flush rate of 1 ml/hour under positive pressure. This device helps prevent clot formation and is especially useful for peripherally inserted central catheters.

Do not rely on the pumps to sound an alarm when an I.V. complication develops. They are fairly efficient at detecting occlusions, but remember, the pump will continue to push fluid when there is no resistance. The I.V. site may be occluded, but if there is a piggyback attached to the pump tubing and the clamp is open, the I.V. solution will be pumped into the piggyback. So, it is good practice to remove (or at least clamp the tubing) the piggyback upon completion of the infusion.

If a line does become clotted, discontinue the line immediately and restart it elsewhere. Immediate discontinuation is necessary to prevent further collection of fibrin on the catheter tip. If this process is allowed to continue, removing the catheter from the vein could dislodge the thrombus and cause an embolus.

Venous spasm

Venous spasm can occur suddenly for various reasons; whatever the cause, it is painful. The patient will typically describe the pain as traveling up the arm, even if the catheter is in the hand.

Venous spasm can be caused by a cold infusate, an irritating solution (such as a hypertonic solution), or a rapid I.V. rate. The latter can best be explained by imagining water going through a garden hose. Water forced with the same pressure through a hose with a ¼″-diameter will have a more piercing stream than water of the same force flowing through a ¾″-diameter hose. If the gauge of the catheter is very small and the I.V. rate is fast, the vein may spasm because a sharp stream of fluid, in a sense, is piercing or stabbing the vein wall.

To treat spasm, apply a warm compress and temporarily decrease the I.V. flow rate. However, the spasm may recur when the rate is reset to the ordered rate. Warm compresses may only delay the inevitable restart of the I.V. line. If a fast rate is ordered, a larger-gauge catheter in a larger vein may be necessary to prevent spasms.

The best way to prevent venous spasm is to promote hemodilution. Choosing a large-bore vein and a small-gauge catheter can reduce the likelihood of venous spasms. Also, be sure the I.V. solution is at room temperature before beginning an infusion.

The anxiety a patient sometimes experiences in anticipation of I.V. therapy can cause a systemic vasospasm, making venipuncture difficult. This is called vasovagal response or attack. Always prepare the patient prior to venipuncture. Allow the patient to breathe calmly and deeply, and discuss concerns to alleviate fears, but do not delay too long. Prolonging the procedure can only increase fear.

If the patient seems overly anxious and identifying an appropriate site is difficult, ask the patient to take deep breaths and place the patient in a supine position. Talk quietly with the patient about something other than needles. Simply using the word needle can cause systemic vasospasm.

Hematoma

Hematoma is another complication that could result from venipuncture or from inadequate pressure applied to veins when the access device is removed. If blood is allowed to escape from the vein, it collects under the skin, causing a bruise. It is common to see extensive bruising on elderly patients' arms because of their thin, delicate veins and skin texture. Applying pressure and elevating the limb is recommended when discontinuing an elderly patient's I.V.

Damage of nerves, tendons, and ligaments

If a patient experiences extreme pain and a feeling of shock during venipuncture, stop the procedure immediately. You may be traumatizing nerves, which could lead to paralysis. The patient may feel numbness and muscle contractions immediately afterward that may continue on and off for hours. Reassure the patient. Explain that the sensation will cease.

If the shocking sensation or numbness develops from an existing I.V. site, consider that the tape or armboard may be too tight. Remove the tape or armboard, and allow the patient time to move fingers and wrist to see if the numbness is caused by the tight tape. It may be necessary to remove the catheter and restart in another location.

SYSTEMIC COMPLICATIONS

Systemic complications that may occur with I.V. therapy include circulatory overload, systemic infection, air embolism, and allergic reactions.

Circulatory overload

Changes in the respiratory system commonly result from fluid imbalances in the body. Onset of respiratory distress, neck vein engorgement, crackles in the lungs, and increased difference between fluid intake and output are common signs of circulatory overload resulting from I.V. therapy.

If a patient receives I.V. fluid faster than the body can distribute and remove the fluid, it will accumulate and cause circulatory overload. If you notice the patient demonstrating signs of overload, immediately raise the head of the bed, administer oxygen, slow the I.V. rate to KVO status, and call the physician. Do not remove the I.V. because you might need it to administer I.V. medications after consulting the physician.

Preventing circulatory overload is of major concern when administering I.V. solutions and medications. Use of I.V. pumps and controllers and rate monitoring devices, especially for elderly, pediatric, and fluid-controlled patients is the first step. Along with that, frequent monitoring is essential—not just for circulatory overload, but for all complications of I.V. therapy.

Systemic infection (septicemia or bacteremia)

Contamination of the I.V. site and I.V. solution are both common sources of systemic infection. Fever, chills, and general malaise may indicate systemic infection. This type of infection can result from poor insertion technique or failure to adequately maintain the I.V. site once the line is placed.

Immunocompromised patients are especially prone to developing septicemia. Severe phlebitis, taping that does not adequately prevent catheter movement, and prolonged indwelling time of the catheter can lead to septicemia.

Blood cultures will be necessary to detect the causative organism and to specify which antibiotic will be needed to treat the infection. It is recommended that the site and device also be cultured. A new I.V. site should be used.

Air embolism

Air from empty I.V. containers that is allowed to enter the patient's vascular system can lead to air embolism. Symptoms include irregular breathing, weak pulse, decreased blood pressure, and loss of consciousness.

If symptoms develop, discontinue the infusion, and do not remove the catheter. Place the patient in Trendelenburg's position. This allows air to enter the right atrium and to dispense it through the pulmonary artery. Administer oxygen, and notify the physician. Thoroughly document the patient's condition and the steps taken to correct the problem.

Prevent air embolism by eliminating air and the potential for air in the I.V. system. Make sure that all ports are plugged, all latex ports are intact (not leaking), and all connections are secure. Prime all tubing before connecting it to the I.V. access device. Use air-eliminating devices and pumps that detect air in the tubing. Make sure that the I.V. containers are not allowed to empty completely. Keep in mind that I.V. solutions are all slightly overfilled, so you can safely throw the I.V. container away when 50 ml or so is still in the container.

Allergic reactions

The body can react to anything that is placed on or in it, including I.V. solutions and medications. An allergic reaction is suspected if a patient develops rashes, unexplained itching, erythema, swelling, wheezing, bronchospasm, neurologic changes, and anaphylaxis.

If the I.V. solution or medication is suspected as the cause of the reaction, stop the solution. Maintain airway, breathing, and circulation

(ABC), as necessary. Notify the physician. Be sure the I.V. remains patent; it likely is to be needed for administering medications to treat the symptoms.

The best way to prevent allergic reactions is by obtaining a thorough history of patient allergies and cross-referencing this information prior to administering any medication. Anticipate using test doses for those who are allergic to similar medications (those in similar pharmacologic classes). It is always important to monitor a patient closely when administering a medication for the first time. Remember, most serious adverse reactions occur within the first 15 minutes of medication administration.

8 ADMINISTERING I.V. MEDICATIONS

The proper preparation and safe administration of medications is of paramount importance in intravenous (I.V.) therapy. As a nurse, you are responsible for knowing the indications, action, dosage guidelines, interactions, and adverse reactions of every drug you administer, regardless of whether it is administered orally, intramuscularly, rectally, or intravenously. When administering I.V. medications, you also must know the correct procedure for preparing drugs and administering them safely to your patient.

This chapter highlights some of the key areas you need to know to safely administer I.V. medications. However, remember that you should always take the time to learn as much as you can about the drugs you administer — before administering them. Your primary sources of information should be the manufacturer's literature (package inserts and labels) and your facility's formulary. Also, keep in mind that there are some handy, affordable, and reliable nurse reference guides available that focus on the type of information nurses need to know to ensure the safe administration of I.V. medications.

INDICATIONS FOR I.V. MEDICATIONS
A physician will prescribe I.V. medications for various reasons. The most obvious reason is that the I.V. route delivers medications directly into the bloodstream, thereby producing an immediate result. This enables the patient to begin building and maintaining adequate drug blood levels quickly to achieve the desired effect. This is also why it is imperative that you have the right medication, prepared in the correct fashion, for the right patient — because, once it is administered, there is no retrieving the medication. It is already doing its job, probably before the entire dose is completely administered.

Other reasons for using the I.V. route include an inadequate or nonfunctioning gastrointestinal (GI) system, an inability to administer the medication by any other route, and the need to control peak serum levels of specific medications.

ACTIONS AND REACTIONS
Although medications are administered to achieve a desired effect, sometimes the desired effect does not occur. Instead, the patient may experience another type of effect — either a side effect or an adverse effect. Side effects are expected or common reactions to a given medication, such as nausea, vomiting, and diarrhea. Adverse effects are unexpected or rare reactions to a given medication, such as rashes, respiratory and cardiac changes, and anaphylaxis.

Any medication has the potential to produce adverse reactions. Such reactions occur more rapidly when the medication is administered intravenously. Most serious reactions from I.V. medications occur within 15 minutes after administration.

If an adverse drug reaction occurs, take the following steps:

1. Stop the medication immediately.

2. Maintain a keep-vein-open I.V. line to allow for the administration of lifesaving medications.

3. Observe the patient closely for changes in respirations and heart rate.

4. Notify the physician. (Never leave the patient alone. Have someone stay with the patient.)

5. Prepare to administer emergency medications. (Have the crash or code cart available.)

6. Monitor the patient's vital signs regularly.

7. Begin cardiopulmonary resuscitation if necessary.

In some cases, adverse drug reactions can be life-threatening. Immediate, knowledgeable action is necessary to save the patient's life. Know all pertinent information about the medications you are giving. Know what to expect and always be prepared for the unexpected.

Once the crisis has passed, be sure to report all adverse drug reactions to the pharmacist, who is responsibile for notifying the Food and Drug Administration (FDA), the federal agency that officially tracks medication issues and problems to ensure safe product administration. Unfortunately, such occurrences are underreported in most facilities.

It is equally important for the pharmacist to question the sudden need for diphenhydramine (Benadryl), epinephrine (Adrenalin), aminophylline (Aminophyllin), or hydrocortisone (Solu-Cortef), because these drugs often are used to treat adverse drug reactions and anaphylaxis. The pharmacist is responsible for compiling this information, which may help provide better reporting of adverse reactions.

DRUG INCOMPATIBILITY

The stability of drugs depends on various elements, including temperature, pH, and combination with other drugs. Incompatibilities occur when two drugs (or a combination of a drug and a solution) become unstable, rendering the medication or solution unsafe to administer in many cases.

- Generally, the higher the temperature, the more unstable most drugs become. For this reason, some medications must be kept at room temperature or refrigerated. Storage of medication at proper temperature typically is addressed in the manufacturer's literature.
- When two drugs are mixed in the same soultion, the more similar the pH, the more compatible the medication.
- Physical, chemical, or therapeutic changes may occur when drugs are improperly combined or put into an incompatible solution.

Physical changes are easiest to detect because they produce visible changes, such as:
- precipitation (settling of insoluble salts)
- leaching (drug is absorbed into container or tubing)
- gas formation (bubbling or foaming)
- a change in the color of solution.

Chemical changes often are difficult to detect. They result in toxic breakdown that causes a loss of activity. The drug is irreversibly degraded.

Therapeutic changes occur when drugs are combined (perhaps intentionally) to cause a specific reaction:
- an antagonistic reaction, in which one drug opposes the action of the other drug
- a synergistic reaction, in which one drug aids the action of the other drug.

Other factors that influence drug incompatibility include:
- the concentration of the drugs in solution
- the volume of the drugs in solution
- the length of time during which the drugs are in contact with one another
- the presence or absence of buffers.

Keep in mind that there is a big difference between mixing two I.V. medications in the same solution and administering them via the same I.V. tubing. Medications that are added together in the same solution obviously will remain in contact longer and have a greater volume and concentration than if they are being administered separately via piggyback. So, when asking the pharmacist about compatibilities, be sure to indicate how you will be giving the medications so that the pharmacist can properly evaluate the various factors discussed above.

I.V. ADMINISTRATION METHODS
I.V. medications can be given in a variety of ways and should be administered slowly. The rate of administration is usually ordered by the physician or recommended by the pharmacist. If in doubt about the rate, follow these safe, simple guidelines:
- For I.V. push, administer 1 ml over 1 minute.
- For I.V. piggyback, administer 50 ml over 30 minutes.

However, as stated earlier, always check the manufacturer's package-insert information or the facility's formulary prior to administering any medication.

I.V. push administration
I.V. push medications are administered directly into the I.V. device or tubing. Such medications should be administered by the nurse only via an intermittent I.V. infusion device or I.V. infusion port. Never use a needle and syringe to inject medication directly into a vein. Doing

so would increase the risk of infiltration and extravasation and therefore is considered unsafe.

An I.V. push should take 3 to 5 minutes to complete, depending on the medication and the amount of solution. Whenever possible, further dilute the medication with normal saline (0.9% sodium chloride) solution to have a 10-ml solution. This provides a more dilute solution, which is less painful, less irritating to the vein, and easier to push slowly with more control. Some medications, such as Valium, cannot be further diluted because of their leaching properties.

When administering medication via I.V. push, make it a habit to always clear the catheter with normal saline solution first. This will ensure that all other drugs, including heparin, have cleared the catheter and tubing, thereby preventing incompatibility reactions. Always remember that any drug in the I.V. bag or bottle also is in the I.V. tubing and must be cleared.

Occasionally, nurses will ask if it is necessary to flush with normal saline solution after giving a medication, even if the catheter will be removed immediately after the medication is administered. The answer is yes, especially when administering medication via an intermittent I.V. infusion device (I.V. lock). This practice will ensure that the patient has received the entire dose and that none of the medication is still in the catheter. Also, even the smallest drop of some medications can cause tissue irritation or damage if allowed to get into the tissue. Flushing the medication through the catheter before removal will prevent the risk of tissue damage. A heparin flush is not necessary prior to removal of the catheter, but a saline flush is always recommended.

I.V. piggyback administration
A piggyback (sometimes called a piggy) refers to the administration of an I.V. medication via an I.V. bag containing 50, 100, 200, or 250 ml of solution through an intermittent I.V. infusion device or the main I.V. tubing. The same principle for preventing incompatibilities exists. It may be necessary to flush the device or tubing with normal saline solution prior to administering I.V. piggyback solutions.

Keep in mind the following points when administering an I.V. piggyback solution:

● A piggyback often is referred to as an intermittent medication infusion because it is not a continuous infusion; rather, the medication is administered intravenously according to a schedule.
● An I.V. piggyback must be hung higher than the main I.V. infusion in order to run. This will allow the main I.V. line to begin following completion of the piggyback. If the piggyback and main infusion hang at similar heights, the main I.V. infusion may back up into the piggyback or the piggyback will not run at all. Be sure to adjust the

rate of the piggyback to the controlled rate of the main I.V. line, or else, upon completion of the piggyback, the main I.V. infusion cannot run freely.

● If the I.V. is attached to an intermittent I.V. device, pay close attention to the time of completion. If the piggyback is allowed to finish and the I.V. device is not flushed immediately, the I.V. catheter could become occluded.

● If an I.V. piggyback is administered via a secondary line, the primary line requires a backcheck valve to prevent the piggybacked medication from flowing into the primary line.

Administration of I.V. medication via a volumetric chamber
Administration of I.V. medication via a volumetric chamber is much like that for an I.V. piggyback. The I.V. solution attached to the volumetric chamber is used as the solution for administering the medication. This method often is used when administering I.V. medications to infants, children, and adults who require strict control over I.V. fluid intake.

The solution in the I.V. bag is allowed to enter the chamber until it holds the desired diluted amount. Then, the pathway between the I.V. solution container and the chamber is closed off. The I.V. medication is added to the chamber via the medication port and set to infuse over the desired amount of time. Once completed, the pathway between the I.V. solution and chamber is opened and a continuous infusion is resumed.

Administration of I.V. medication via a continuous infusion
Medication added to large volumes of I.V. solution and administered without interruption is called continuous infusion. Heparin, aminophylline, insulin, and total parenteral nutrition (TPN) are a few examples of continuous medication infusions. These infusions should be regulated very carefully with an infusion pump or controller to guarantee proper flow rate.

Note: Never interrupt continuous infusions to give an intermittent I.V. medication. They must be kept at a continuous rate to achieve proper therapeutic effects.

PRECAUTIONS FOR I.V. ANTIBIOTIC ADMINISTRATION
I.V. antibiotics probably are the most commonly administered group of I.V. piggyback medications. Take the following precautions when administering any I.V. infusion, especially when administering any antibiotic.

● Check for patient allergies because cross-sensitivity may occur. For example, penicillin-sensitive patients should not receive cephalosporins. If the physician prescribes one of these medications, a test dose should be given to evaluate patient tolerance.

- Assess for early symptoms of allergic reaction, including rash, fever, urticaria, migraine, and GI disturbances.
- Watch closely for decreased urine output and rising blood urea nitrogen and serum creatinine levels because decreased renal function may result (especially with aminoglycosides).
- After prolonged use, monitor for superinfection caused by overgrowth of nonsusceptible organisms.
- Follow up on culture and sensitivity studies to determine susceptibility of the causative organism to the prescribed antibiotic.
- Ensure that the patient is well hydrated. This helps transport the medication throughout the body and helps excretion of the medication.
- Watch for outdated medications of any kind because nephrotoxicity can result from administration of antibiotics that have expired.
- Make sure that the patient receives the entire dosage ordered to ensure maximum effect.
- Take steps to prevent vein irritation. The Intravenous Nurses Society recommends rotating sites every 48 hours to prevent vein irritation; the Centers for Disease Control recommends rotating sites every 48 to 72 hours.
- Check the manufacturer's package insert for stability data when diluting vial contents for I.V. infusion. Each medication differs in stability after dilution.
- Always check with the pharmacist or the package insert for complete information on incompatibilities of any two (or more) medications to be mixed in solution or administered through the same tubing. Remember that not all reactions resulting from mixing incompatible medications are obvious.

9 BLOOD TRANSFUSIONS

This chapter focuses on administering blood and blood products, which can be unnerving to the inexperienced nurse. Even many experienced nurses prefer not to administer blood products because of possible adverse reactions, such as depression, anxiety, and anaphylaxis.

Currently, many patients feel anxious about receiving blood transfusions because they fear contracting acquired immunodeficiency syndrome (AIDS), which is transmitted through blood and body secretions. The fear of contracting hepatitis B from blood transfusions used to be the major concern, but it largely has been replaced by the fear of AIDS.

When participating in a blood transfusion, allow the patient to express concerns and offer reassurances. Encourage open communication. Explaining the procedure and educating the patient about how blood is screened will help alleviate some anxiety. Explain to the patient that all donor blood is labeled according to ABO and Rh groupings and is tested extensively before routine transfusion for hepatitis B surface antigen; for antibody to human immunodeficiency virus (HIV), which causes AIDS; and for syphilis and other sexually transmitted diseases (using rapid plasma reagin [RPR] card test and the Venereal Disease Research Laboratory [VDRL] test).

PREPARATION

Blood type is determined by the presence of A, B, and O, and Rh groups in the blood. Crossmatching will determine compatibility between donor and recipient. Blood typing and crossmatching is essential prior to administration of blood.

A donor's blood patient is crossmatched to guarantee that the blood is compatible with the patient's blood. Blood samples from the patient and donor must be studied to identify the type and the Rh factor of their blood prior to administration. An error in typing and crossmatching can be fatal.

Blood type is determined by the ABO group. The presence of antigens on the red blood cells determines the type of blood. The Rh factor is also an important part of typing and crossmatching blood. Rh antibodies do not develop without immunizing stimulus. Red blood cells with D antigens are called Rh-positive, and red blood cells without D antigens are called Rh-negative. If the person with Rh-negative blood receives Rh-positive blood, hemolysis occurs.

ADMINISTERING A TRANSFUSION

Three main objectives for administering blood or blood products are:
- replacing and maintaining blood volume
- replacing and maintaining oxygen-carrying capacity of the blood (by supplying red blood cells)
- replacing and maintaining coagulation properties (by supplying the coagulation factors found in platelets and plasma).

Various types of blood components may be transfused. The patient's condition determines the type needed. (For more information, see *Comparing Blood Components,* pages 108 to 111.)

The nurse responsible for transfusion therapy must adhere to specific rules for safe administration. These include:
- Check the physician's orders. Be sure what blood product is required.
- Make sure that patient or family has signed a written, informed consent form before administering a blood transfusion.
- Check the patient's blood identification with another nurse. Avoiding mistaken identity is imperative. It is recommended that the patient's name is spelled and repeated and the unit identification numbers verbalized and repeated. Avoid interruptions and check closely.
- Inspect the blood before administering it to avoid infusing hemolyzed, clotted, or contaminated blood. Look for discoloration and clumps. This could indicate contaminated blood.
- Maintain proper technique. Use sterile technique for spiking the bag. Use precautions, such as gloves, to prevent exposure to blood.
- Observe the patient closely. Early detection of the signs and symptoms of a reaction is important.

Check and recheck the blood (with another nurse) and the patient identification band to ensure that you are infusing the blood that has been crossmatched for that particular patient. Evaluate the patient before, during, and after administering blood and blood components. Reactions to blood or blood products can occur 5 minutes to several hours after an infusion begins. To determine baseline data, vital signs (temperature, pulse, and respiration) should be obtained just before transfusion.

Stay with the patient for the first 15 minutes of the transfusion, then assess vital signs again. Watch closely for reactions during this time because most transfusion reactions occur within the first 15 minutes. Vital signs assessment should be repeated 1 hour after therapy begins and on completion of the transfusion.

Administering cold blood could cause hypothermia and may be fatal to the patient. It may be necessary to administer blood via a blood warming device. This device provides a constant temperature between 89.6° F and 98.6° F (32° C and 37° C). Use of such a special device requires in-service education for normal operation and for trouble-

(Text continues on page 111.)

COMPARING BLOOD COMPONENTS

The chart below highlights the indications and nursing considerations for various blood components used in transfusions.

Component	Indications	Nursing considerations
Whole blood Complete (pure) blood	• To restore blood volume in patients with hemorrhage, trauma, or burns • To treat symptomatic anemia with large fluid volume deficit	• ABO-identical match is necessary. • Use straight-line or Y-port I.V. set. • For massive loss, infusion should be given as fast as the patient can tolerate it. Maximum infusion time is 4 hours. • Know that labile coagulation factors deteriorate within 24 hours. • Associated risks include hepatitis, circulatory overload, and allergic or febrile reactions. • Contraindicated when patient has condition responsive to specific blood components.
Packed red blood cells (RBCs) Same RBC mass as whole blood with 80% of the plasma removed	• To restore or maintain oxygen-carrying capacity of the blood • To correct anemia and blood loss resulting from surgery • To increase RBC mass	• ABO compatibility is necessary. • Use straight-line or Y-port I.V. set. • For massive loss, infusion should be given as fast as the patient can tolerate it. Maximum infusion time is 4 hours. • Associated risks include hepatitis, allergic reactions, and febrile reactions. • Generally, RBCs have the same oxygen-carrying capacity as whole blood, but without the hazards of volume overload. • Using packed RBCs avoids potassium and ammonia buildup that sometimes occurs in the plasma of stored blood. • Contraindicated in patients with pharmacologically treated anemia or coagulation factor deficiency.
Leukocyte-poor blood Same as packed RBCs, except 70% of leukocytes are removed	• Same as packed RBCs • To prevent febrile reactions from leukocyte antibodies • To treat immunosuppressed patients	• ABO compatibility is necessary. • Use straight-line or Y-port infusion set. May require a Pall filter (40-micron filter) for hardspun, leukocyte-poor RBCs. • Infusion should be given over 1½ to 4 hours. • Other considerations same as for packed RBCs.

COMPARING BLOOD COMPONENTS *(continued)*

Component	Indications	Nursing considerations
White blood cells (leukocytes) Whole blood with all the RBCs and 80% of the supernatant plasma removed	• To treat a patient with life-threatening agranulo-cytosis (granulocyte count usually under 500/mm³) who is not responding to antibiotics	• ABO compatibility is necessary. Preferably, should also be human leukocyte antigen (HLA) compatible but not necessary unless patient is HLA-sensitized from previous transfusions. • Use straight-line set with standard in-line blood filter. • Dosage is 1 unit daily for 5 days or until infection resolves. Infusion should be given over 1 to 2 hours. • Infusion induces fever and chills; associated risks include hepatitis and allergic reactions. • Administer an antipyretic if fever occurs, but do not discontinue transfusion. Flow rate may be reduced for patient comfort. • Give transfusion in conjunction with antibiotics to treat infections. • Contraindicated when bone marrow function recovery is necessary to sustain life.
Platelets Platelet sediment from RBCs or plasma, resuspended in 30 to 50 ml of plasma	• To treat thrombocyto-penia caused by de-creased platelet production, increased platelet destruction, or massive transfusion of stored blood • To treat acute leukemia and bone marrow aplasia • To restore platelet count preoperatively in patient with a platelet count of 100,000/mm³ or less	• Cross-typing for ABO compatibil-ity is not necessary, but is preferred for repeated transfusions. Rh matching also is preferred. • Use a component drip administra-tion set without a microaggregate filter; infuse 100 ml over 15 minutes. • Associated risks include hepatitis and allergic and febrile reactions. • Patients with a history of platelet rejection require premedication with antipyretics and antihistamines. • Avoid administering platelets when patient has a fever. • A blood platelet count may be or-dered 1 hour after transfusion to determine platelet transfusion incre-ments. • Usually contraindicated for pa-tients with conditions of accelerated platelet destruction, such as idio-pathic thrombocytopenia purpura, or drug-induced thrombocytopenia.

(continued)

COMPARING BLOOD COMPONENTS *(continued)*

Component	Indications	Nursing considerations
Fresh frozen plasma (FFP) Uncoagulated plasma separated from RBCs	• To expand plasma volume • To treat postoperative hemorrhage or shock • To correct an undetermined coagulation factor deficiency • To replace a specific coagulation factor when that factor alone is not available • To correct coagulation factor deficiencies resulting from hepatic disease	• Cross-typing is same as for platelets. • Use a straight-line I.V. set and administer rapidly (approximately 10 ml/minute). Maximum infusion time is 2 hours. • Large-volume transfusions of FFP may require correction for hypocalcemia. Citric acid in FFP binds with calcium. • Associated risks include hepatitis, allergic or febrile reactions, and circulatory overload. • Contraindicated for patients with conditions responsive to specific concentrates.
Albumin 5% (buffered saline); albumin 25% (salt-poor) Small plasma proteins prepared by fractionation of pooled plasma	• To replace volume in treatment of shock caused by burns, trauma, surgery, or infection • To replace volume and prevent marked hemoconcentration • To treat hypoproteinemia (with or without edema)	• ABO matching is not necessary. • Use a straight-line I.V. set and infuse according to patient's condition and response. • Adverse reactions (fever, chills, nausea) are rare. • Albumin should not be mixed with protein hydrolysates or alcohol solutions. • Commonly given as a volume expander until crossmatching for whole blood is complete. • Contraindicated in patients with severe anemia and is administered cautiously in patients with cardiac and pulmonary diseases because of the risk of congestive heart failure from circulatory overload.
Factor VIII (cryoprecipitate) Cold, insoluble portion of plasma recovered from FFP	• To treat hemophilia A and von Willebrand's disease • To control bleeding associated with factor VIII deficiency • To replace fibrinogen or factor VIII • To treat hypofibrinogenemia	• ABO compatibility not necessary, but preferable. • Use the manufacturer-supplied administration set; administer with a filter. • Standard dose recommended for treatment of acute bleeding episodes in hemophilia is 15 to 20 units/kg. May require rapid infusion and frequently repeated doses.

COMPARING BLOOD COMPONENTS *(continued)*		
Component	**Indications**	**Nursing considerations**
Factor VIII (cryoprecipitate) *(continued)*		Half-life of factor VIII (8 to 10 hours) necessitates repeat transfusions every 8 to 10 hours to maintain normal levels. ● Contraindicated in patients with unidentified coagulation defects. ● Associated with hepatitis, allergic reactions, and febrile reactions.
Factors II, VII, IX, and X complex (prothrombin complex) Lyophilized, commercially prepared solution drawn from pooled plasma	● To treat congenital factor V deficiency and other bleeding disorders resulting from an acquired deficiency of factors II, VII, IX, and X	● ABO and Rh matching is not necessary. ● Use a straight-line I.V. set; dosage is based on desired level and patient's body weight. ● Associated with a high risk of hepatitis. ● Coagulation assays are performed before administration and periodically during treatment. ● Contraindicated in patients with hepatic disease resulting in fibrinolysis and in those with intravascular coagulation who are not undergoing heparin therapy.

shooting problems. Never use incubators or microwave ovens to warm blood; doing so can cause hemolysis. (See *Blood Transfusion Tips,* pages 112 and 113, for more information.)

Electronic monitoring devices are recommended to ensure adequate infusion time whenever possible. However, the user of such equipment must be familiar with the device to ensure proper usage and to know how to troubleshoot problems when alarms sound. Gravity-flow administration is not recommended because of the possibility of free flow and inadequate rate of infusion. Close observation of the I.V. site is necessary to ensure that infiltration does not occur.

Nurses also should have a working knowledge of the different types of tubing and filters needed when administering blood products. Blood tubings often have a 170-micron filter that is used to remove any clumps or blood clots. It may be necessary to increase the filtering capabilities by using a micropore or microaggregate filter. These filters, which have a pore size of 20 to 40 microns, are used to remove leukocytes from the blood. Immunosuppressed and pediatric patients often benefit from using these filters.

BLOOD TRANSFUSION TIPS

1. Follow the facility's policies and procedures for transfusion therapy.

2. Hang the blood within 30 minutes after receiving it from the blood bank. It cannot be reissued if kept out of the controlled environment of the blood bank, where it is refrigerated at 33.8° to 42.8° F (1° to 6° C).

3. If blood is obtained from the blood bank, but not hung immediately, return it to the blood bank for proper temperature control.

4. Use a blood warming device to administer blood to a patient with cold agglutinins and to any patient receiving a massive transfusion. Cold blood may produce cardiac effects and general hypothermia.

5. *Use normal saline solution (0.9% sodium chloride) only.* Blood should not be infused with hypotonic or hypertonic solutions. Hypotonic solutions cause water to invade the red blood cells until they burst, resulting in hemolysis. Hypertonic solutions dilute the blood cells, causing them to shrink.

6. *Never administer medication* with blood transfusions.
  • Bacterial contamination is a hazard because blood hanging in a warm room offers a good medium for bacterial growth; therefore, to maintain a sterile infusion, do not penetrate ports with needles from piggyback infusions.
  • Pharmacologic incompatibilities may exist.
  • The drugs may be administered too slowly to achieve therapeutic levels.

7. *Use a filter* during infusion. A sterile pyrogen-free filter of 170 microns is required. (Follow package directions for best results.) Tubing used for blood transfusions is usually Y-tubing, which allows normal saline solution and blood to be readily infused.

8. Remember, the larger the vein, the faster the transfusion can be administered.

9. The rate of transfusion depends on the patient's condition. Most patients can tolerate one unit of blood transfused over 1½ to 2 hours. A patient with congestive heart failure or pulmonary edema will require a much longer period for transfusion.

10. *Infuse blood completely within 4 hours* of removing it from the blood bank to avoid the danger of bacterial growth and hemolysis. Set the infusion to run over 2 hours unless otherwise specified by the physician. This gives you time to correct any problems that may arise.

11. After the transfusion is complete, be sure to document the volume of the blood component infusion. Check the bag, and note the volume for accuracy.

12. Remember, standard procedure calls for blood to be infused through an 18G or 20G cannula for adults. For practical purposes, however, a 22G cannula already inserted in a patient should not be removed to infuse blood, especially if the patient has limited venous access. The infusion will require close monitoring. It may need to be run slightly faster and the bag elevated higher to maintain movement through the cannula because of the viscosity of the blood, but it will be sufficient. Also, remember that because a 20G or 22G cannula is sufficient to infuse blood to a child, a 22G cannula may be sufficient for transfusing most blood components to adults. However, do not use a 22G cannula when transfusing blood via a pump because hemolysis may occur.

BLOOD TRANSFUSION TIPS *(continued)*

13. Most importantly, be sure the right patient gets the right blood. Check the blood with another nurse. Do not take this final check lightly. Read each letter and number aloud, and verify by repeating what you see, not what you hear. Errors can easily be made if both nurses do not take the time to check thoroughly.

14. Completely fill out the paperwork associated with administration of blood.

15. Obtain baseline vital signs, which are extremely important, before beginning the infusion. A fluctuation of one degree in the temperature is an indication that the patient may be having a reaction to the blood. If a transfusion reaction occurs, initiate treatment immediately.

The number of tubing and filter changes is usually dependent on the manufacturer. However, it is good practice to use the same tubing for up to two units of blood. Microaggregate filters may only be designed to infuse one unit of blood. Always take the time to read the packaging of the tubing and filter to guarantee proper use.

Transfusion reactions

A transfusion reaction refers to an antigen-antibody reaction that occurs in the recipient due to an incompatibility between red blood cell antigens and antibodies in which the antibody combines with the red blood cell possessing the corresponding antigen. Signs and symptoms of transfusion reaction include:
- chills
- fever
- flushing
- burning sensation along the vein
- lumbar or flank pain
- oozing of blood at the injection site and from surgical areas
- chest pain
- shock
- hemolysis (urine changes color).

If any of these signs or symptoms occur, begin treatment immediately:
- Stop the transfusion by closing the clamp closest to the patient.
- Run normal saline solution to maintain vein patency.
- Notify the physician. (Follow orders appropriate to the symptoms exhibited by the patient.)
- Notify the laboratory about the transfusion reaction.
- Label the unused blood and tubing as "Blood transfusion reaction," and send them to the laboratory for analysis.
- Label the first-voided urine specimen as "Blood transfusion reaction," and send it to the laboratory.

(For more information, see *Blood Transfusion Reactions,* pages 114 and 115.)

BLOOD TRANSFUSION REACTIONS

The chart below identifies the causes, signs and symptoms, and usual treatment for blood transfusion reactions requiring prompt treatment.

Reaction	Cause	Signs and symptoms	Treatment
Febrile reaction	• Antileukocytic antibodies in the recipient are directed against the donor's leukocytes	• Usually occurs late in or after the transfusion. • Characterized by flushed face, palpitations, cough, feeling of tightness in chest, increased pulse rate, chills, and fever (up to 104° F [40° C], not lasting more than 8 hours).	**1.** Stop the transfusion and run normal saline (0.9% sodium chloride) solution. **2.** Notify the physician immediately. **3.** Initiate symptomatic treatment immediately.
Allergic reaction	• Allergies or hypersensitivities to certain drugs in donor blood	• Urticaria and hives occasionally accompanied by chills and fever. • Severe reactions include fever, wheezing, shortness of breath, and anaphylactic shock.	**1.** Stop transfusion. **2.** Notify physician immediately. **3.** Administer antihistamines. **4.** Administer epinephrine or steroids in severe cases.
Delayed hemolytic reaction	• Immune antibody response to foreign antigen in a previous transfusion	• Hemolysis, mild anemia, and increased serum bilirubin levels occuring 2 to 11 days after transfusion.	**1.** Notify physician. **2.** Test to detect direct Coombs' antibody.
Circulatory overload	• Blood transfused too rapidly • Whole blood given to patient with increased volume	• Headache, tightness in chest, flushed feeling, back pain, chills, fever, cyanosis. • Congestive heart failure, as characterized by shortness of breath, dyspnea, orthopnea, cyanosis, diaphoresis, jugular vein distention, bibasilar crackles, and dependent edema. • Pulmonary edema, as characterized by increased blood pressure and cerebrovascular pressure, diffuse crackles, shortness of breath, rapid breathing.	**1.** Stop transfusion. **2.** Elevate patient's head. **3.** Notify physician immediately. **4.** Phlebotomize, if necessary. **5.** Administer diuretics, if necessary.

BLOOD TRANSFUSION REACTIONS *(continued)*

Reaction	Cause	Signs and symptoms	Treatment
Air embolism	• Can occur when large amounts of air enter the bloodstream, causing tenacious bubbles in the blood to become lodged in the pulmonary capillaries	• Characterized by cyanosis, dyspnea, shock, and cardiac arrest.	**1.** Stop transfusion. **2.** Position patient on left side with head down. (This traps air in right atrium, preventing it from entering the pulmonary artery. The pulmonic valve is kept clear until the air can escape gradually.) **3.** Notify physician immediately. **4.** Treat symptoms immediately.
Hypothermia	• Occurs from massive replacement of cold blood	• Characterized by chills, lowered body temperature, peripheral vasoconstriction, and cardiac arrest.	Warm blood to 95° F (35° C) with automatic blood warmer during rapid replacement.

Delayed reactions also may occur up to 160 days after transfusion, and AIDS may present many years later. Some common delayed reactions include:

• *Hepatitis B* (occurs 50 to 160 days after transfusion) has been reduced greatly due to the detailed screening of donors. Blood is tested for the hepatitis B surface antigen (HBsAg). This testing, along with detailed questioning of voluntary donors, has contributed to the decrease in the transmission of hepatitis B resulting from blood transfusion. However, for patients receiving blood products, the risk of hepatitis B still is higher than for any other blood-borne pathogen, including AIDS.

• *Syphilis* is nearly eliminated from the list of delayed reactions for the patient receiving blood due to serologic testing. Refrigeration has a spirocheticidal effect; therefore, stored blood provides less risk than fresh blood products.

• *Malaria* is a disease for which no practical screening method is available. Donors who have taken malaria prophylaxis or have been treated for malaria within the last 3 years are deferred.

• *AIDS*, caused by HIV, has been a source of great fear since the early 1980s. In 1985, a test for the presence of the HIV antibody has been used to protect the nation's blood supply. However, it is not definitive of the disease, only of exposure to the disease. An incubation period of 6 to 24 months exists. Donors are deferred according to sexual activity, drug history, and history of blood transfusions.

● *Cytomegalovirus (CMV)*, which can exist in healthy adults, can be fatal for immunosuppressed patients. People with CMV exhibit fatigue, weakness, adenopathy, and low-grade fever. Many facilities screen blood for CMV.

Autologous transfusion

Donor blood is not the only way to receive blood products. A patient may donate blood at the blood bank prior to having surgery to ensure that he or she receives only his or her own blood if necessary postoperatively. The blood is donated in the patient's name and marked for autologous transfusion. This greatly reduces the risk of blood transfusion reactions. The patient must have a physician's order to give blood for this reason.

10 CHEMOTHERAPY

Chemotherapy is a medication regimen given to a patient who has been diagnosed as having a specific illness. This chapter deals with patients receiving chemotherapy for cancer and the medications (commonly called antineoplastic agents) used to treat it. The drugs may be given orally or parenterally; however, this discussion will focus on drugs given parenterally. Keep in mind that the oral drugs may have the same adverse reactions as the parenteral ones.

Patients undergo extensive testing to diagnose their condition before any chemotherapy is given. The oncologist may then treat the patient in one or all of the following ways:

- through surgery to explore the condition and remove the cancer in part or in whole
- through radiation to decrease the size of the tumor, stop its growth, or shrink it so that the cancer is contained enough to be operable
- through chemotherapy, using antineoplastic agents to systemically destroy the cells involved in cancer growth and prevent the spread of the disease. Chemotherapy may be given for treatment or palliation.

Depending on the type of cancer and its course, all of these steps may be necessary. Surgery allows for firsthand visualization of the cancer and for removal of all or part of the cancer involved. Surgery also may be necessary after radiation or chemotherapy to see exactly how the cancer responded to treatment. Radiation therapy, a successful treatment for decreasing the growth of cells, is used when a tumor or mass is present. It also may be used to reduce the size of a tumor before surgery.

An oncologist will order chemotherapy for a patient when the systemic approach provides the best means for reducing the number of cancer cells. Depending on the cancer involved, the oncologist will order one or a combination of antineoplastic agents and prescribe dosages to be administered to the patient.

Patients need to be educated about their specific type of cancer and the treatment they will receive. Also, they should be informed that chemotherapeutic drugs are toxic and can cause adverse reactions. Nurses should be aware that these drugs must be handled carefully.

HOW CHEMOTHERAPY WORKS

All cells go through a series of steps, called the cell cycle, to reproduce. Antineoplastic agents effectively destroy cells at specific stages of development during the cell cycle.

The cell cycle

The cell cycle is divided into five distinct phases:

● G_1 — During this postmiotic phase, enzymes are produced that are necessary for deoxyribonucleic acid (DNA) synthesis. The time frame for this phase is highly variable.

● S — During this phase, DNA synthesis occurs. Duration is 10 to 20 hours.

● G_2 — During this short, premiotic phase, ribonucleic acid (RNA) is synthesized and the miotic spindle is made. Duration is 2 to 10 hours.

● M — During this short mitotic phase (duration is ½ to 1 hour), the cell actually divides, and the process is accomplished in five stages:
— Prophase: the nuclear membrane disappears, the cell begins to break down, and chromosomes begin to clump
— Metaphase: chromosomes line up in the middle of the cell
— Anaphase: chromosomes segregate to the centrioles
— Telophase: cell division occurs, resulting in two daughter cells
— Interphase: resting stage (long phase).

● G_0 — During this resting phase, the cell is not participating in division. Duration is highly variable.

● G_1 and G_0 are in equilibrium with each other.

(For more information, see *The Cell Cycle,* page 119.)

Cancer cells can grow anywhere in the body and do not follow normal cell reproduction. Tumors grow slowly until they become vascular, then their growth accelerates. The oncologist may order a single medication or a combination of medications to destroy cells during specific stages of development.

Antineoplastic agents

Most antineoplastic agents disrupt DNA synthesis. They have their greatest effect on rapidly dividing cells, such as the cells of the mucous membranes and bone marrow. Chemotherapy affects both normal cells and cancer cells, but whereas normal cells can repair themselves, cancer cells are less able to do so. The goal of chemotherapy is to eradicate the cancer cells while minimizing the toxic effect on the normal cells.

Antineoplastic agents are classified into two groups: cell-cycle-specific (CCS) drugs and cell-cycle-nonspecific (CCNS) drugs. CCS drugs act only at a specific phase of the cell cycle, or they are dependent on the cell cycle. They are usually given in multiple doses to patients with bulky tumors. CCNS drugs act independently of the cell cycle, acting on several or all cell cycle phases, and work best on slow-growing tumors.

Antineoplastic agents are commonly grouped into six pharmacologic classifications: alkylating agents; antineoplastic antibiotics; antimetabolites; natural plant (vinca) alkaloids; hormonal antineoplastic agents;

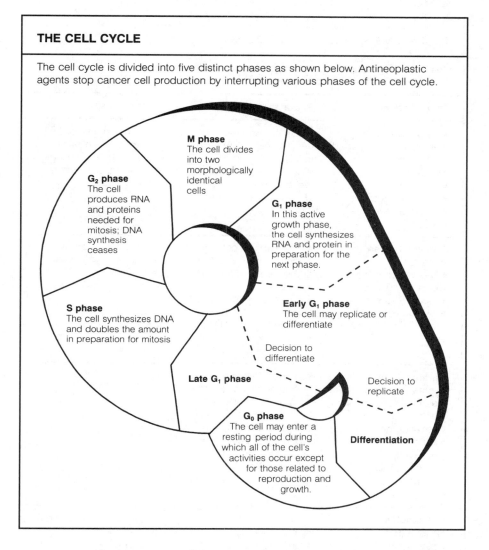

THE CELL CYCLE

The cell cycle is divided into five distinct phases as shown below. Antineoplastic agents stop cancer cell production by interrupting various phases of the cell cycle.

M phase
The cell divides into two morphologically identical cells

G_2 phase
The cell produces RNA and proteins needed for mitosis; DNA synthesis ceases

G_1 phase
In this active growth phase, the cell synthesizes RNA and protein in preparation for the next phase.

S phase
The cell synthesizes DNA and doubles the amount in preparation for mitosis

Early G_1 phase
The cell may replicate or differentiate

Decision to differentiate

Late G_1 phase

Decision to replicate

G_0 phase
The cell may enter a resting period during which all of the cell's activities occur except for those related to reproduction and growth.

Differentiation

and nitrosoureas. (For more information, see *Comparing Antineoplastic Agents,* pages 120 and 121.)

To ensure maximum cancer cell kill, combination chemotherapy may be needed. This treatment attempts to destroy cells at various cycles by using drugs from two or more pharmacologic categories. For example, doxorubicin, cyclophosphamide, and vincristine may be given for ovarian cancer.

DRUG PREPARATION

The safest method of antineoplastic drug preparation is under a laminar flow hood with vertical ventilation, vented to the outside. This prevents exposure to the harmful chemicals from drug aerosolization.

COMPARING ANTINEOPLASTIC AGENTS

The following chart provides a comparative view of the characteristics and toxic effects of some of the most commonly used antineoplastic agents.

Type of agent	Characteristics	Toxic effects
Alkylating agents • altretamine • busulfan • chlorambucil • cisplatin • cyclophosphamide • dacarbazine • melphalan	• Interfere with deoxyribonucleic acid (DNA) replication • Cell-cycle-nonspecific (affect both resting and dividing cells)	• Affect the hematopoietic system, gastrointestinal (GI) system, and gonads • Cause tissue necrosis
Antimetabolites • cytarabine • fluorouracil • mercaptopurine • methotrexate • thioguanine	• Produce fake compound in cell that replaces normal protein required for DNA synthesis • Cannot produce nucleotides and therefore no ribonucleic acid (RNA) • Attack mostly during S phase of cell cycle	• Affect bone marrow, central nervous system, and GI system • Cause myelosuppression
Hormonal antineoplatic agents • adrenal suppressants • androgens • antiandrogens • antiestrogens (tamoxifen) • corticosteroids • estrogens • progestins	• Interfere with binding of normal hormones to receptor proteins; manipulate hormonal levels and alter hormonal environment • Decrease growth fractions of cancer cells • Therapy is usually palliative and not cytotoxic or curative	• Lack cytotoxicity
Antineoplastic antibiotics • bleomycin • dactinomycin • daunorubicin • doxorubicin • mitomycin • plicamycin	• Bind with DNA to inhibit synthesis of DNA and RNA • Cell-cycle-nonspecific	• Affect GI, renal, and hepatic systems • Affect bone marrow • Cause tissue damage (except bleomycin)
Natural plant (vinca) alkaloids • vinblastine • vincristine • vindesine	• Bind to substances necessary for miotic spindle formation, thereby preventing cell division • Attack during M phase of cell cycle	• Affect GI, central nervous, and peripheral nervous systems • Cause tissue damage (except VePesid) • Cause myelosuppression

COMPARING ANTINEOPLASTIC AGENTS *(continued)*		
Type of agent	**Characteristics**	**Toxic effects**
Nitrosoureas • carmustine (BCNU) • semustine (methyl CCNU) • lomustine (CCNU) • streptozocin	• Interfere with DNA replication • Cell-cycle-nonspecific (affect both dividing and resting cells)	• Cause suppression of hematopoiesis • Affect GI system (severe nausea and vomiting) • Cause thrombocytopenia
Miscellaneous agents • etoposide • hydroxyurea • L-asparaginase • procarbazine • cisplatin • paclitaxel	• Not fully understood; do not conform to other classes	• Produce various effects

When preparing medications for administration and during their actual administration, it is essential to wear powder-free, disposable surgical gloves. Some guidelines call for double gloves in instances where gloves may not be of the best quality and prolonged contact with the chemical is likely. It is important to change the gloves hourly and immediately if they become torn or punctured. Powder-free gloves are recommended because the powder increases the particulate level in the work area and absorbs contamination from the chemicals in the work area.

Protective gowns should always be worn. Ones that are made of lint-free, low-permeability fabric and that close in the front and have long sleeves and tight cuffs are recommended to protect the skin and clothing from contamination.

A plastic, punctureproof, shatterproof, closable hazardous waste container should be available wherever chemotherapy agents are prepared and administered. Such a container is used for disposal of contaminated needles, syringes, filters, tubings, and intravenous (I.V.) containers without exposure to the immediate environment.

If working with a medication that is in an ampule, gently shake down the medication in the ampule and wrap gauze around the neck of the ampule before breaking it in a direction away from your body. This will prevent aerosolization.

When preparing to administer I.V. chemotherapeutic agents, consider the following points:

• Prepare the medications without interruptions and always take your time.

- Prime the administration set in the work area prior to injecting the medication into the I.V. container; this prevents priming in a less-controlled environment.
- Use luer-lock fittings wherever possible, to prevent spills due to disconnection.
- Be sure the I.V. bag is properly labeled, along with a warning about its contents, so that it is handled properly.
- Transport the medication in a sealable plastic bag to reduce the chances of accidental exposure to the toxins.

PATIENT PREPARATION AND CARE

Treatment with chemotherapy begins after the following considerations have been completed:

- The patient's consent has been obtained.
- The patient's condition has been determined by a baseline physical examination as performed by a physician according to the Karnofsky scale — an evaluating system used to summarize a patient's general condition during the course of illness that uses percentages to quantify the patient's activity level at that point.
- The tumor growth pattern has been recognized.
- The drug regimen has been matched with the patient's condition.

A good baseline determination of the patient's physical condition is important, because the nurse needs it to monitor the therapeutic response. The physician also must consider basic cell chemistry when choosing the drugs for each patient. With combination chemotherapy, he must consider that each drug has a different dosage range to achieve maximum cancer cell kill while allowing the patient to maintain normal body functioning with minimal toxicity.

Scheduling a patient's treatment depends on two factors: the tumor growth pattern and the patient's recovery time. Giving intermittent doses will allow time for adequate recovery from the toxic effects of chemotherapy on the hematopoietic, integumentary, and gastrointestinal systems. The proper timing of treatment ensures that the tumor cells do not have adequate time to redevelop.

Destroying a maximum number of cancer cells with each treatment is the goal of chemotherapy. However, it is important to remember that the total number of cancer cells to be treated should be fewer with each treatment. Also remember that these agents are potentially toxic to the patient and the nurse.

Patients receiving chemotherapy have various experiences. Each patient reacts in a different way. Before the treatment begins, patients should be warned about the potential adverse reactions. (For more information, see *Adverse Reactions to Chemotherapy,* page 123.)

Frequently, cancer patients depend on nurses for emotional support and physical care. Allow patients to verbalize their feelings. Do not

ADVERSE REACTIONS TO CHEMOTHERAPY

Adverse reactions result from the action of antineoplastic agents on all rapidly dividing cells. Commonly affected cells include those of the bone marrow, mucous membranes, gastrointestinal tract, and hair follicles.

COMMON REACTIONS

Nausea and vomiting can occur immediately upon administration of the drug and up to 3 days after treatment; they may occur with anticipation of treatment.
Myelosuppression is perhaps the most dangerous reaction. The bone marrow is responsible for housing the precursor or stem cells for the major blood components: red blood cells, white blood cells, and platelets. Damage to any of the stem-cell population will result in a decrease in the number of mature cells found in the peripheral blood. Because chemotherapeutic agents are toxic to these stem cells, the patient's blood will show a decrease in mature, fully functioning blood cells, leaving the patient anemic and susceptible to other illnesses, especially infection.

In some instances, low blood levels are a contraindication to administering I.V. chemotherapy. A physician may wait to see the laboratory test results before ordering the medication regimen.
Hair loss occurs because the cells of hair follicles divide rapidly and they also are affected by chemotherapeutic agents. The effects of hair loss, especially for women, can be emotionally devastating. Explaining the potential for hair loss prior to initiating chemotherapy helps both male and female patients deal with the loss. It probably is best to help the patient deal with hair loss as a reality, instead of focusing on prevention of hair loss. Provide information about hair and scalp care. Stress that protecting the scalp from sun and cold is very important. If the patient decides to wear a wig, encourage the purchase of a "soft-cap" wig to prevent scalp irritation.

OTHER REACTIONS

Weakness and fatigue can be caused by the drug or by excessive nausea and vomiting.
Mood swings commonly present as depression: the patient typically is afraid of being sick and of dying.
Restlessness, chills, and fever can be very frightening to a patient; they may indicate drug intolerance or possible infection.
Allergic reactions to chemotherapeutic agents sometimes occur. Common reactions include urticaria, agitation, dyspnea, hypotension, facial edema, abdominal cramps, laryngospasm, stridor, rash, pruritus of the hands and feet, and loss of consciousness. Although deaths linked to allergic reactions have been reported, most patients recover after treatment is stopped. Early assessment and treatment (commonly with epinephrine or glucocorticoids) are essential in ensuring a positive outcome.

isolate patients unless infection is suspected or their laboratory work indicates myelosuppression. Family and friends should be encouraged to help with providing care.

It is understandable that the patient fears the possibility of death. It is necessary to offer support honestly, but with hope. Allow the patient to speak openly about death, but remember that cancer is not always terminal.

Be alert for the signs of grieving. According to Kubler-Ross's stages of dying, the patient may experience any or all of the following stages: denial, anger, bargaining, depression, and acceptance.

A cancer patient is under tremendous stress and may need quiet and rest. Be aware the the patient may choose to have no visitors while in the hospital and, especially, while receiving treatment. Honor the patient's wishes about visitors, and remember that his or her frame of mind is important. Every patient responds differently to cancer and chemotherapy. Listen to the patient and try to make him or her as comfortable as possible.

Include the patient in the treatment plan. Consider the patient's previous experiences with chemotherapy as well as the patient's concerns about how chemotherapy may have affected family members and friends who have undergone similar treatments. Allow the patient to express these concerns. Explain that all patients react differently to the same medication, but that some similarities exist, depending on the drug therapy used.

Hair loss is a major concern for most cancer patients who will receive chemotherapy. Offer the use of soft rubber tourniquets, inflatable scalp pressure cuffs, and ice caps to decrease circulation to the scalp; these devices help prevent or minimize hair loss. However, never offer false hope. These devices, although helpful for some, have not been useful for most. Encourage the patient to deal with the reality of hair loss.

Commonly, nurses and patients fear the drug itself. It is important to be aware of the effects of these drugs and use them safely. Irritants can lead to phlebitis and can cause pain and burning of the vein.

Preventing vein trauma is a central issue that nurses have to contend with when administering I.V. chemotherapy. It is essential that the patient have a patent, healthy I.V. line. A peripheral catheter should be inserted just prior to administration of chemotherapeutic agents. Never use a catheter that has been previously placed and has had time to infiltrate or irritate the vein wall.

Many new materials are used in catheter manufacturing, and they should be considered when administering chemotherapy. Previously, stainless steel needles were recommended over Teflon for the administration of various agents. Recently, over-the-needle catheters have become popular in chemotherapy administration. In most cases, they can be well placed without the fear of vein wall puncture resulting from needles.

Take the time to find out what material the catheter is made of, and thoroughly review the literature about the ordered medication. Pay close attention to the recommendations for cannula types. For example,

Taxol reacts with Teflon catheters, causing a red irritated vein within hours after initiation. Vialon catheters do not seem to cause the same problem with Taxol.

If using a surgically implanted device for chemotherapy administration, all of the above points still apply. Keep in mind that visualizing infiltrations is more difficult. Catheter patency and vein integrity are essential for any catheter placement. Extravasation can be extremely painful for the patient and the nurse; if the chest wall is involved, it can be extensive and devastating.

When administering chemotherapy via an implanted port, be sure to thoroughly flush with a normal saline and heparin flush. The noncoring needle should be well flushed before its removal from the port so that none of the agent is allowed to come into contact with the tissue when it is withdrawn from the port. Always heparinize prior to removing the noncoring needle so that the catheter contains some heparin.

ADMINISTRATION OF ANTINEOPLASTIC AGENTS

When administering antineoplastic agents, you must take special precautions to safeguard youself and your patient from contamination with these toxic agents. Always wear protective equipment, and keep in mind the following tips.

Venipuncture

- Ask for assistance with venipuncture if access to a peripheral vein proves difficult. A healthy vein is very important in preventing extravasation.
- Avoid accessing a vein that may flow into previously used areas. Extravasation from these sites is possible.
- Avoid using major veins, such as the antecubital fossa. Distal veins are preferred because they allow successive proximal venipuncture.
- Avoid using extremities with impaired circulation (caused by mastectomies, lymphedema, immobilized fractures, invading neoplasms, phlebitis, and varicosities, for example).
- Avoid using leg veins because the potential for thrombophlebitis exists.
- Avoid using bruised, inflamed, or sclerosed veins. Damaged veins increase the risk of extravasation.
- Alternate venipuncture sites when administering chemotherapy to allow previous veins to heal.
- Use a small-gauge catheter for administration. The Intravenous Nurses Society recommends using the smallest gauge that will properly infuse the ordered medication.
- Always run an isotonic (normal saline, 0.9% sodium chloride) solution in a freshly inserted I.V. catheter to verify vein integrity prior to drug administration.

During administration

- Have emergency drugs and extravasation kits available at all times when administering I.V. chemotherapy.
- Keep the entire arm or accessed area visible during administration, and watch closely for adverse reactions and signs of infiltration.
- Always follow the ordered protocol. Chemotherapy medications are commonly prescribed in a specific sequence. Be sure to premedicate the patient as ordered, and follow the ordered sequence to ensure a therapeutic effect.
- Be aware that there are different theories about when to administer irritants and vesicants. Some believe that the vesicant should be given first when the vein is at its healthiest; some believe that it should be administered last.
- Check for a blood return every 2 or 3 minutes when administering an agent by I.V. push. When giving an infusion, monitor the I.V. site every hour for blood return and signs of infiltration.
- Use an electronic monitoring device to infuse all I.V. chemotherapeutic medications.
- Be sure to flush the catheter well with normal saline solution between doses of I.V. push chemotherapeutic agents.
- When in doubt about vein integrity, discontinue the infusion and initiate a new site.

After administration

- Flush the catheter well with normal saline after administering a chemotherapeutic agent, before removing the catheter, to ensure that none of the agent is on or in the catheter. Even the smallest amount of some agents can cause tissue damage.
- Document the medications given, the date and time of administration, the site used, the condition of the site before and after treatment, and any unusual or untoward reaction.
- Keep in mind that patients receiving certain cytotoxic agents may excrete high concentrations of the drug or its metabolites. Handle blood, urine, feces, and vomitus with protective equipment (especially gloves), and guard against splashing. Most agents are fully excreted within 48 hours.
- For incontinent patients, use disposable pads; place all soiled pads in a hazardous waste container. Separate and label linens that have been contaminated with cytotoxic agents or body fluids after antineoplastic drug administration.

Disposal and accidental exposure

- Consider all cytotoxic agents as hazardous, and handle them accordingly.
- Check your institution's protocol for disposal of hazardous wastes. Hazardous waste can be incinerated or placed in a licensed sanitary landfill specifically designated for hazardous waste.

- Use appropriate containers for disposing of needles, syringes, vials, ampules, and I.V. solution containers. Such containers should be sealable, punctureproof, leakproof, and clearly labeled and should be readily available where agents are prepared and administered (including the patient's room).
- Dispose all protective equipment used in preparing and administering cytotoxic drugs in hazardous waste containers.
- Educate all employees involved in preparation and administration of cytotoxic drugs about safe handling and disposal of these agents.
- Intervene immediately if accidental exposure occurs:
  1. Remove the gloves and gown.
  2. Wash exposed skin with soap and water. Do not use germicidal agents.
  3. If drug comes in contact with eyes, flush eyes for at least 5 minutes with isotonic solution and obtain medical assistance as soon as possible.
- Document the event in the employee's record, including drug, type, concentration, and approximate volume of exposure.

Spill management
- Have instructions and materials for spill management readily available in any area where cytotoxic agents are prepared or administered.
- Follow the guidelines established by the Occupational Safety and Health Administration for keeping the following equipment available in kit form for immediate use:
  — Two pairs of powder-free surgical gloves
  — One disposable gown made of lint-free, low-permeability fabric with a closed front, long sleeves, and elastic cuffs
  — One pair of shoe covers
  — One pair of chemical splash goggles
  — One dust/mist respirator mask
  — Two sheets (12″ × 12″) of absorbent material
  — One 250-ml and one 1-liter spill-control pillow
  — One scoop to collect glass fragments
  — Two large cytotoxic waste disposal bags.
- Restrict access to the area of the spill.
- Contain the spill (a priority).
- Place glass fragments in a punctureproof, sealable container.
- Take care to prevent aerosolization of the chemicals.

EXTRAVASATION
Cytotoxic agents are classified as either vesicants or irritants. A vesicant is any agent capable of causing blistering and tissue damage. An irritant is any agent capable of causing achiness, itching, feeling of tightness, or phlebitis either at the injection site or along the vein path. An inflammatory reaction or a flare reaction (a local reaction manifested

by pruritus and red blotches following the course of a vein and subsiding within 30 to 60 minutes) also may occur following administration of a vesicant or irritant.

The leakage of a vesicant or an irritant into the subcutaneous tissue is called extravasation. Probably the most frightening problem (next to anaphylaxis) that a nurse can witness when administering chemotherapy, extravasation can cause pain, necrosis, and sloughing of tissue. Although the literature indicates that the incidence of extravasation is only 6%, it can cause the patient serious disfigurement and diminish his or her quality of life. The treatments are controversial.

The extent of tissue damage from extravasation depends on the amount of drug given and the concentration of the extravasated drug. The mechanism of injury with vesicant drugs is not completely understood. The chemotherapeutic drug associated with the highest risk for tissue damage is doxorubicin hydrochloride (Adriamycin RDF, Adriamycin PFS), which destroys tissue because it is retained in the tissue for weeks, thus resulting in damage to viable cells and delayed wound healing.

Veins are located between the dermis and subcutaneous fat. The fat protects the tendon, muscles, and nerves from infiltrated and extravasated solutions. Full-thickness loss of skin can result if a vesicant is allowed to exit the vein. Consequently, because of the decreased amount of subcutaneous fat, the dorsum of the hand and the joints are not used for the administration of chemotherapeutic agents.

When vesicants are to be a part of the chemotherapeutic regimen, a long-term central venous access device should be considered. This type of device is less likely to cause infiltration; however, extravasation is still a possibility and, because of its location, can be even more devastating.

Preventing extravasation
Prevention of extravasation is essential. The following points should always be considered prior to administration of all cytotoxic drugs, especially vesicants.

- Assess vein integrity. Assess the skin and integrity of the area surrounding the catheter. (For more information, see *Assessing for Peripheral Extravasation and Other Reactions*, page 129.)
- Ensure vein visibility. Be sure that the area around the catheter is visible during the entire chemotherapy administration.
- Ensure catheter stability. Be sure that the catheter is stabilized at all times, especially during chemotherapy administration.
- Administer drug via an infusing I.V. side port. Administration of cytotoxic drugs via an administration port on a continuous I.V. infusion is recommended. This helps verify vein integrity before and during the infusion, and helps dilute the medication as it is administered.

ASSESSING FOR PERIPHERAL EXTRAVASATION AND OTHER REACTIONS

The chart below lists the parameters to be assessed when identifying whether the patient has experienced extravasation, vein irritation, or a flare reaction.

Assessment parameter	Extravasation	Vein irritation	Flare reaction
Blood return	Inability to obtain blood return; however, may still be present in some cases	Usually present	Usually present
Pain	Severe pain or burning lasting minutes to hours, eventually subsiding; usually occurs when drug is being given, at the needle site	Aching and tightness along the vein	No pain
Redness	Blotchy redness may occur at needle site	Full length of vein may be reddened or darkened	Immediate blotches or streaks along vein as drug is given; usually subsides within 30 minutes with or without treatment
Swelling	May occur at needle site either immediately or hours later	Not likely	Not likely
Ulceration	Develops insidiously, usually 48 to 96 hours after drug administration	Not likely	Not likely
Other	Change in quality of infusion; increased resistance; local tingling; sometimes sensory deficits appear as delayed manifestations	None	Itching

● Provide patient teaching. Inform the patient to report any pain, burning, stinging, or itching at the I.V. site or along the vein path.
Antineoplastic drugs given over long periods, such as continuous slow drips of fluorouracil and cisplatin, should be observed routinely, at least every 2 hours. If a drug is a vesicant (known to cause tissue

damage), it should be observed hourly. When observing these infusions, always assess the:

- condition of the I.V. site
- ability to obtain an adequate blood return
- patient's tolerance of treatment
- patient's sensation of the I.V. site
- flow rate.

And, as always, make sure to document your observations completely.

Treating extravasation

Every facility should have a procedure for treating extravasation, as immediate treatment is always necessary. If extravasation occurs, evaluate the site, keeping in mind the following:

- Which drug is involved?
- How much of the drug has leaked into the tissues?
- How long was the drug in contact with the tissues?

Although a definitive antidote has not been defined for extravasation involving doxorubicin, mechlorethamine, or vinca alkaloids, the local injection of steroids, administration of sodium bicarbonate, and topical application of dimethyl sulfoxide (DMSO) have been reported to be effective. Keep in mind that most extravasations never progress beyond mild local irritation, even when antidotes have not been given. According to current research, the best treatment for doxorubicin extravasation is to immediately remove the I.V. line and apply ice to the site for 30 minutes to 10 hours and intermittently for up to 7 days (Groenwald, 1993).

If mechlorethamine, a nitrogen mustard extravasates, administer isotonic sodium thiosulfate 1 g/10 ml. Mix 4 ml of 10% sodium thiosulfate with 6 ml of sterile water for injection (1/6 molar solution) to achieve an isotonic sodium thiosulfate solution. Inject the isotonic sodium thiosulfate through the existing I.V. line and administer subcutaneously into the extravasated site, according to your facility's protocol or the physician's orders. Apply cold compresses to the affected area. Delayed treatment is ineffective.

If vinca alkaloids (such as vincristine, vinblastine, or vindesine) extravasate, hyaluronidase dissolved in saline solution should be injected liberally into the extravasation site immediately after removal of the I.V. tubing. Heat is then applied to activate the hyaluronidase. Do not use cold applications and steroids, as they increase the skin toxicity of vinca alkaloids.

Nurses cannot order treatment for extravasation, but they are often the first to recognize that extravasation has occurred. Prompt treatment is essential. The presence of an extravasation kit with the necessary equipment would help expedite the treatment if an extravasation occurs.

It is also important to closely watch the site of surgically implanted venous access devices when administering I.V. chemotherapy. Although infiltration and phlebitis are less likely to occur in these devices, they may occur. Watch for burning, pain, or swelling around the device, in the area of the chest, neck, back, or in the clavicular area.

Surgical interventions may be necessary when severe necrosis results. Debridement and repair may be necessary. Recovery is a long process that may require physical rehabilitation.

It cannot be stressed enough that nurse education is mandatory. Nurses must be aware of the potential hazards of handling and administering chemotherapeutic agents. They also must be fully aware of the potential venous complications and how to deal with them quickly and responsibly.

11 PARENTERAL NUTRITION

This chapter discusses parenteral nutrition, a form of nutrition that is delivered intravenously to maintain a proper metabolic state, maintain positive nitrogen balance, and promote tissue synthesis. A solution containing amino acids, carbohydrates, fats, vitamins, electrolytes, and trace elements is used.

When illness or surgery prevents a patient from eating and metabolizing food, parenteral nutrition may be necessary. Depending on the type of therapy ordered, nutritional support solutions will be given either through a peripheral device (this type of nutritional support is called peripheral parenteral nutrition [PPN]) or a central venous access device, including a peripherally inserted catheter whose tip lies in a central vein (this type of nutritional support is called total parenteral nutrition [TPN]).

Indications for parenteral nutrition

TPN may be administered to a patient with any of the following conditions:
- a debilitating illness lasting longer than 2 weeks
- limited or no oral intake for longer than 7 days, such as in cases of multiple trauma, severe burns, or anorexia nervosa
- after a 10% or greater loss in pre-illness weight
- serum albumin level below 3.5 g/dl
- poor tolerance of long-term enteral feedings
- chronic vomiting or diarrhea
- continued weight loss despite adequate oral intake
- gastrointestinal (GI) disorders that prevent or severely reduce GI absorption, such as bowel obstruction, Crohn's disease, ulcerative colitis, short-bowel syndrome, and bowel fistulas
- inflammatory GI disorders, such as pancreatitis and peritonitis
- excessive nitrogen loss resulting from wound infection, fistulas, or abscesses
- renal or hepatic failure.

Patients who do not need to gain weight yet need nutritional support may receive PPN for as long as 2 to 3 weeks. PPN is commonly used to:
- maintain or restore fluid and electrolyte balance
- maintain homeostasis before and after surgery
- help a patient meet minimum calorie and protein requirements.

This therapy also may be used as an adjunct to oral or enteral feedings for a patient needing to supplement a low calorie intake. PPN may be given to a patient who is unable to absorb enteral therapy.

PARENTERAL NUTRITION SOLUTIONS

Parenteral solutions are prepared according to individual patient needs as prescribed by a physician. The specific solution will depend on the type of parenteral nutrition and the patient's status. These solutions may be administered either peripherally or through a central venous access device.

Parenteral nutrition solutions consist of the following components:

- dextrose (supplies most of the calories)
- amino acids (supply protein)
- fats (supply a concentrated energy source)
- electrolytes (replace needed electrolytes depending on the patient's condition)
- vitamins (ensure normal body functioning and optimal use of nutrients)
- micronutrients (promote normal metabolism)
- water (maintains fluid balance depending on the patient's condition).

Other specialized solutions are available for use with patients who have cardiac, renal, or hepatic disorders or who are experiencing severe bodily stress. (For more information, see *Basic Parenteral Nutrition Solutions*, pages 134 and 135.)

Peripheral parenteral nutrition

If the solution is delivered peripherally, the solution is usually a nearly isotonic mixture of glucose, amino acids, fat, vitamins, minerals, and electrolytes. The concentration of glucose usually does not exceed 10% in the peripheral formula, in which case the solution is then slightly hypertonic. A greater concentration could cause serious vein trauma, burning of venous tissue, and pain.

Although the risk of sepsis is reduced because the peripheral access devices are changed more frequently, strict asepsis and care during PPN administration is essential. Complications that may develop with the peripherally administered solutions include thrombophlebitis and local tissue damage (if infiltration occurs).

Total parenteral nutrition

Solutions administered centrally are very hypertonic solutions. TPN solutions are administered via central venous access devices, preferably into the superior vena cava, so that the solutions (which can have an osmolarity five times that of plasma) can be infused into a large vessel, allowing for rapid dilution (usually a dilution factor of at least a thousand).

Use of a large vessel to administer TPN decreases the risk of thrombophlebitis. However, the risk of sepsis is much greater than via the peripheral route because of the greater concentration of glucose in the solution and the easy access of bacteria into a major vessel.

Catheter sepsis is of great concern when accessing the central venous system. Organisms normally found on the patient's skin and the nurse's

BASIC PARENTERAL NUTRITION SOLUTIONS

The chart below highlights some of the common solutions used for parenteral nutrition.

Solution	Indications	Formula contents	Breakdown of contents	Caloric content
Standard central solution	● Acceptable for most patients who require parenteral nutrition	● 500 ml dextrose 50% ● 500 ml amino acids 8.5%	Contents for each 1,000 ml of solution: ● 42.5 g amino acids ● 250 ml dextrose ● 6.5 g nitrogen	1,020 kcal/liter (850 kcal as non-protein calories)
Low-carbohydrate solution	● Used for patients who cannot tolerate high glucose load or who show evidence of carbohydrate overfeeding ● Designed to administer fat emulsions to compensate for reduced carbohydrate calories	● 500 ml dextrose 30% ● 500 ml amino acids 8.5%	Contents for each 1,000 ml of solution: ● 42.5 g amino acids ● 150 g dextrose ● 6.5 g nitrogen	680 kcal/liter (510 kcal as non-protein calories)
Cardiac solution	● Used for patients with volume intolerance; it is a balanced amino acid protein source in a hypertonic dextrose solution	● 500 ml dextrose 70% ● 500 ml amino acids 10%	Contents for each 1,000 ml of solution: ● 50 g amino acids ● 350 g dextrose ● 7.65 g nitrogen	1,390 kcal/liter (1,190 kcal as non-protein calories)
Renal solution	● Used for patients with acute tubular necrosis who can tolerate moderate fluid administration and do not have severe hyperkalemia or other electrolyte disturbances	● 500 ml dextrose 70% ● 250 ml amino acids 5.4%	Contents of each 750 ml of solution: ● 12.75 g amino acids ● 350 g dextrose ● 1.6 g nitrogen	1,240 kcal/750 ml (1,190 kcal as non-protein calories)

BASIC PARENTERAL NUTRITION SOLUTIONS *(continued)*				
Solution	Indications	Formula contents	Breakdown of contents	Caloric content
Hepatic solution	• Used for patients with chronic liver disease (solution may be altered slightly depending on the grade of disease)	• 500 ml dextrose 50% • 500 ml branched-chain, enriched amino acids 8%	Contents of each 1,000 ml of solution: • 40 g amino acids • 250 g dextrose • 6 g nitrogen	1,010 kcal/liter (850 kcal as non-protein calories)
Stress solution	Used for critically ill or traumatized patients and in those with sepsis or in hypermetabolic states in the immediate postinjury period; for added calories, lipid emulsion may be added	• 250 ml dextrose 70% • 750 ml branched-chain, enriched amino acids 6.9%	Contents of each 1,000 ml of solution: • 52 g amino acids • 175 g dextrose • 7.3 g nitrogen	903 kcal/liter (595 kcal as non-protein calories)
Peripheral solution	• For patients who have no central venous access or in whom central venous acces is contraindicated • Used for 3 to 5 days of nutrition support in patients whose oral intake is not certain	• 500 ml dextrose 10% • 500 ml general purpose amino acids 7%	Contents of each 1,000 ml of solution: • 35 g amino acids • 50 g dextrose • 5.5 g nitrogen	310 kcal/liter (170 kcal as non-protein calories)

hands are commonly responsible for catheter-related sepsis. Strict hand-washing protocols, asepsis, and catheter maintenance and security are essential to prevent catheter-related sepsis.

A physician may request additives, such as heparin and hydrocortisone, in the solution to prevent central vein thrombosis. There are differing opinions as to whether antibiotics should be administered directly to the TPN solution or via a secondary infusion line. Adding antibiotics directly is thought to decrease nursing time, conserve venous access, and control fluid volume. However, potential risks include catheter contamination and central vein thrombosis. Catheter manipulation and use of intermittent administration of antibiotics further increase these risks.

TPN maintains lean body mass, promotes tissue function, and maintains nitrogen balance. Usually, the body burns up its supply of fat and carbohydrates for energy. During an illness, if fat and carbohydrates are unavailable, the body will break down protein from the muscles. This process occurs when a patient suffers starvation or has a low carbohydrate intake. Deamination of the body's tissue proteins provides the body with glucose (this process is called gluconeogenesis) to lay the groundwork for metabolic functions. The fuel for organ function comes from ketoacids provided by fatty acids obtained from the body's adipose tissue. TPN given to debilitated patients will supply them with the necessary nutrients (plus protein) to prevent muscle wasting by sparing protein supplies.

An adult requires 1 to 1.5 g of protein/kilogram of ideal body weight to spare body proteins. The nutritional and caloric needs of each patient are determined by height, weight, age, body temperature, physical condition before admission, presence of infection, and ability to digest and absorb nutrients.

Patients receiving regular I.V. fluids will develop fluid overload before they are supplied with sufficient calories and volume nutrients. Therefore, a more concentrated solution, such as TPN, is required. TPN can supply as much as 300 to 5,000 calories per 1,000 ml bag.

Total nutritional admixtures (TNA, 3-in-1 solutions) are TPN solutions with lipids and other additives combined in one container. Little literature is available on the use of these solutions. Opinions differ as to their safety and effectiveness. Stability of the fat emulsion may be altered by the pH of the solution. Electrolytes and amino acids may alter the pH significantly enough to increase or decrease the stability of the fat emulsion.

Using TNA or 3-in-1 solution can increase the pH of the solution because of the addition of fat emulsion, which can cause precipitation of calcium and phosphate salts. Conversely, the addition of calcium can result in immediate emulsion breakdown. (Fischer, 1991)

Fat (lipid) emulsions

If supplemental calories are required, fat emulsions will be ordered along with the dextrose solution. No more than 60% of the total calories to be administered should be fat. This infusion can be added to the TPN line below the filter and set to infuse via its own infusion device.

It is recommended that a test dose of lipids be administered prior to administration of the solution. Administration of 1 ml/minute over a 30-minute period is suggested to ensure that patient can tolerate the solution.

ADMINISTERING PARENTERAL NUTRITION

Depending on whether the patient requires maintenance or replenishment of nutrition, either PPN or TPN will be used. Generally, TPN is used to replace nutrients in markedly malnourished and severely catabolic patients to boost their daily caloric intake. PPN usually is used for maintenance therapy, for patients who have had nothing by mouth for more than 3 days, and for those who are not expected to eat again for the next 10 to 14 days.

Parenteral nutrition can be given either continuously or cyclically. With continuous parenteral nutrition, the patient receives the infusion over a 24-hour period, beginning at a slow rate that is gradually increased as ordered by the physician. With cyclic therapy, the patient receives 1,000 to 2,000 calories overnight and the balance of nutrients orally the next day. Home-care parenteral nutrition programs have boosted the popularity of cyclic therapy, which also may be used to wean the patient from TPN.

Administering PPN

Using a combination of amino acid-dextrose solution and lipid emulsion, PPN supplies the patient's full caloric needs without the risks associated with central venous access. Because a PPN solution has a lower tonicity than a TPN solution, a patient receiving PPN must be able to tolerate large volumes of fluid.

Caring for the patient receiving a PPN infusion involves the same steps as for any patient receiving a peripheral I.V. infusion, including maintaining the solution, tubing, dressings, I.V. site, and infusion devices.

Administering TPN

TPN solutions must be infused into a central vein, using one of the following devices: a peripherally inserted catheter whose tip lies in a central vein, a central venous catheter, or an implanted vascular access device. Long-term therapy requires either a long-term central venous catheter (such as a Hickman, Broviac, or Groshong catheter) or an implanted port (such as the Infuse-A-Port or Port-A-Cath).

Mixing the ordered formula is a procedure that must be performed using sterile technique because the glucose concentration is a great medium for bacterial growth. Use of a laminar flow hood to ensure that the air in the working area is as clean as possible decreases the risk of solution contamination.

Filters are added to the infusion line to remove particulate matter and bacteria from the solution before it reaches the patient. The use of add-on or in-line filters is recommended. A 0.22-micron filter is recommended for solutions without fat emulsion. If administering a 3-in-1 solution (TPN with lipids added), a 1.2-micron filter should be used. Although the 1.2-micron filter will remove candidal organisms, yeasts, and fungi, it is not considered a particulate filter.

TPN solutions should be started and discontinued gradually according to the concentration of dextrose. Solutions with a final concentration of 15% to 25% dextrose should be started at a rate of 40 ml/hour (note that renal and cardiac formulas should begin at a rate of 30 ml/

hour because of their higher dextrose concentration). Then, the rate is adjusted 20 ml/hour/day to meet the caloric needs of that patient. Be sure to follow the physician's order closely, and monitor the patient's blood sugar level carefully for hyperglycemia. If the patient develops an elevated blood sugar level of greater than 200 mg/dl, do not advance the rate; keep in mind that a supplemental dose of insulin may be necessary to control the elevated blood sugar level. The blood sugar values should be discussed with the physician immediately. Changes in the rate and administration of insulin should be done only under physician's orders. NEVER stop the infusion or decrease the rate drastically because this may result in a hypoglycemic incident.

Equally important is the technique for changing the I.V. tubing and caring for the infusion site. Good hand-washing and sterile technique are required to prevent sepsis. Remember, instruct the patient to keep his or her face turned away from the site during routine care of the central line. (See Chapter 3, I.V. Equipment, for more information on central lines.)

The concentration of the TPN solution can influence the route of administration. The solution must be compatible with the route or painful vein irritation can develop. A large-caliber, rapid-blood-flow vein should be used to infuse the hypertonic solution. Hemodilution helps to dilute the concentrated solution to a more isotonic state.

After insertion of the central venous access device, the site must be cleaned and an occlusive dressing must be applied. An antimicrobial ointment may be applied to the insertion site for the patient's protection against microorganisms and to prevent pulling of air into the skin and venous opening.

Patients receiving a TPN infusion should be monitored closely. The use of an electronic infusion device is recommended; however, the device should not take the place of the nurse. Visualization of the site and the rate of infusion is still essential to prevent complications. If the device has a pressure setting, be sure to use the low and medium settings for peripheral infusions and the high settings for central lines only. Using the high setting on a peripheral vein could cause infiltration, which can lead to cellulitis, phlebitis, or extravasation.

The use of an electronic infusion device also is important because the rate of infusion must be consistent. Never play "catch up" or "slow down" to keep on time. A change of more than 10% of the ordered rate can cause one of the following conditions:

- a too-rapid rate. Hyperglycemia will result, causing osmotic diuresis in which the patient will secrete excess glucose. If severe enough, intractable seizures, coma, and death can result.
- a too-slow rate. Hypoglycemia will result. The serum blood glucose level will drop below 50 mg/100 ml and the patient will not receive adequate caloric and nitrogen benefits.

For these reasons, monitoring a patient's excretion of glucose is essential. Testing glucose and acetone levels in the urine should be done every 6 hours; maintaining strict fluid intake and output and keeping a calorie count also are important. Monitor weight daily and assess vital signs every 6 to 8 hours. Because monitoring the fluid and electrolyte status also is crucial, testing should include osmolarity as well as determinations of phosphate, magnesium, blood glucose, blood urea nitrogen, creatinine, and triglyceride levels on a regular basis (according to physician's order).

Other laboratory values that should be monitored are provided below along with their normal levels:

- serum albumin level   3.5 to 5.5 g/dl
- serum transferrin   250 to 410 mg/dl
                             (for child, 350 to 450 mg/dl)
- lymphocyte count   1,500 to 3,000/mm³

Monitoring the albumin level in the blood helps to establish the severity of malnutrition. The following abnormal levels indicate the degree of severity:

3.0 to 3.5 g/dl = mild malnutrition
2.5 to 3.0 g/dl = moderate malnutrition
below 2.5 g/dl = severe malnutrition.

A low serum albumin shows prolonged protein deprivation without acute nutritional changes.

Serum transferrin reflects protein malnutrition. The following abnormal levels indicate the degree of severity:

150 to 250 mg/dl = mild protein depletion
100 to 150 mg/dl = moderate protein depletion
below 100 mg/dl = severe protein depletion.

The total lymphocyte count in the blood falls when a patient is suffering from protein malnutrition. The following abnormal levels indicate the severity of depletion:

1,200 to 1,500/mm³ = mild protein depletion
800 to 1,200/mm³ = moderate protein depletion
below 800/mm³ = severe protein depletion.

Evaluating the patient's laboratory values along with the patient's condition is important. Equally important is observing and caring for the I.V. line from I.V. fluid container to tip of the catheter. Although aseptic technique is used when the catheter is inserted, maintaining an antibacterial environment when the infusion line is in place is crucial.

I.V. line maintenance is critical when administering TPN. To change the dressing, don gloves and remove the old dressing carefully to avoid disturbing the sutures and catheter placement. This is a good time to examine the site. Note the length of the catheter from the exit site to the hub. It is a good idea to chart an approximate length to ensure the catheter's position for future reference. Also, examine the site for tubing kinks, leaks, redness, drainage, and skin irritation.   After removing the dressing, change gloves. A sterile pair is necessary to clean and dress the skin. Clean the site with an antiseptic solution, allowing the solution to remain in contact with the skin for at least 30 seconds. Remember to clean from the center, moving outward. Observe the condition of the patient's skin, and apply the dressing. Benzoin and Skin Prep help protect the skin and secure the dressing. Use paper tape to prevent skin tearing and allergic reactions to adhesive. The dressing must be occlusive to prevent contamination. Transparent dressings or sterile gauze and tape also are appropriate dressing materials.

Keep in mind that all transparent dressings are not alike. Review the manufacturer's literature to identify which dressing is best suited to the patient's needs. Some dressings simply allow evaporation of moisture and prevent entrance of bacteria. The OpSite IV3000 actually pulls moisture to the surface of the skin, then allows evaporation.

Use of transparent dressings is controversial. Always consider the patient; pulling and tugging the skin can cause abrasions and microabrasions, and the movement of the catheter causes in-and-out movement (much like a piston), which can predispose the the patient to infection. It is best to use a dressing that secures the catheter to prevent movement for a long period of time and to allow for continuous visualization of the site.

Remember to secure the catheter in a position that will prevent accidental dislodging and patient discomfort. Ask the patient to move the affected limb or the neck (depending on the I.V. line position) to check whether the catheter is comfortable and secure. Keep in mind the patient will have to live with that site for a while after the procedure has been completed.

The Intravenous Nurses Society has set the following standards for TPN administration:

- Final filtration and electronic infusion devices should be used.
- All solutions exceeding 10% dextrose or 5% protein in content must be administered via a central line.
- Solutions consisting of 10% dextrose or lower and 5% protein or lower may be administered via a peripheral line.
- Use of peripheral TPN should be limited to 7 to 10 days because this type of solution will not provide adequate nutrition over an extended period.
- Parenteral nutrition solutions should be used immediately after preparation or refrigerated.

- Once hung, parenteral solutions must be infused or discarded within 24 hours.
- Always verify the catheter tip placement before administering TPN solution.
- When therapy is ending, the rate should be decreased gradually to avoid hypoglycemia.
- All parenteral nutrition solutions should be filtered with a 0.2-micron filter except when lipid emulsion is added to these solutions, at which time a 1.2-micron filter should be used.
- No medications should be added to these solutions once they are hung.
- Solutions should be prepared in a pharmacy under a laminar flow hood to maintain sterility of the solution.
- The nurse's responsibility prior to administration includes — but is not limited to — reviewing the patient's height, weight, nutritional status, diagnosis, and current laboratory values.

Remember that the health of a patient receiving TPN is already compromised. Therefore, you must use aseptic technique when setting up the TPN infusion to maintain a sterile environment. Otherwise, sepsis can occur. (For more information, see *Administering Total Parenteral Nutrition*.)

ADMINISTERING TOTAL PARENTERAL NUTRITION

Follow the general guidelines below to ensure safe total parenteral nutrition (TPN) administration.

GENERAL CONSIDERATIONS

- Never administer TPN without a physician's order.
- Ensure that the solution was prepared by the pharmacy and mixed under sterile conditions. Check that the solution is properly labeled with the date of preparation, date of expiration, and list of additives.
- Never insert additives to the solution outside of the pharmacy.
- To ensure asepsis, make sure that you have received the proper training and have demonstrated competence before administering TPN to any patient.
- Never infuse anything other than TPN in the I.V. line in which TPN is infused.

BASIC EQUIPMENT

- Solution: Always check against the physician's order to make sure that you are using the correct solution, and verify the patient. Also check to see that the solution is free of visible contaminates.
- Monitoring device: Use a controlling device or I.V. pump for precise infusion of the amount ordered.
- Tubing: Be sure that it is appropriate for the monitoring device and ordered rate.
- Final filter: If the tubing does not have an in-line filter, a final filter is necessary.
- Gloves: Always wear gloves to ensure asepsis.   *(continued)*

ADMINISTERING TOTAL PARENTERAL NUTRITION *(continued)*

PREPARING FOR TPN ADMINISTRATION

• Infuse only normal saline (0.9% sodium chloride) solution until the cannula X-ray confirms placement; this minimizes the risk of infiltration.
• Obtain a chest X-ray to confirm cannula placement and rule out the possibility of pneumothorax.
• Remove the solution from the refrigerator ½ hour before hanging the solution to prevent complications associated with infusing a too-cold solution, such as shock and vasospasm.
• Compare the physician's order with the solution to ensure that the proper additives have been included.
• Check the solution for signs of contamination by observing for color, clarity, and particulate matter.

ADMINISTERING TPN

• Wash your hands, applying at least 10 seconds of friction to help prevent the spread of infection and cross-contamination.
• Assemble the equipment, keeping all junctions sterile. Use sterile gloves to decrease the possibility of contamination.
• Add a final filter to secure all connections.
• Prepare the solution container for spiking.
— If the TPN solution is in a bottle, expose the tubing port and listen for release of a vacuum upon removing the rubber stopper. Absence of a vacuum release may indicate that the solution is contaminated.
— If the TPN solution is in a bag, expose the port for spiking.
• Spike the solution container, keeping the spike and port sites sterile.
• Prime the tubing to prevent air embolism.
• Connect the tubing to the cannula hub.
— When administering TPN via a peripheral line, use aseptic technique as with insertion of any peripheral I.V. line.
— When administering TPN via a central venous catheter, turn the patient's face away from the site and connect the line while the patient exhales. If possible, have the patient hold his or her breath during the connection to decrease the possibility of airborne contamination and air embolism.
— When administering TPN through a surgically implanted device, such as a Hickman or Groshong catheter, clamp the catheter before connecting the TPN tubing to prevent air embolism.
• Set the flow rate.
• Check all connections to ensure that they are secure. Taping the connections may help prevent disconnection of the tubing.
• Secure the tubing to prevent manipulation of the dressing and I.V. site and to prevent contamination.
• Label the tubing with the date and your initials to ensure proper tubing changes.
• Document the procedure in the patient's record, noting the date, time, and patient's tolerance of the procedure.

ADMINISTERING TOTAL PARENTERAL NUTRITION (continued)

MAINTAINING ASEPSIS

- Change all lipid infusion sets every 24 hours; remove the set upon completion of lipid administration to prevent line contamination.
- Maintain a clean, secure dressing to prevent airborne and general contamination.
- Avoid contaminating the site with oral or tracheal secretions.
- Use a bib or plastic linen drape to cover the central venous access site. A transparent dressing is also helpful.
- Monitor vital signs closely because temperature elevation, hypotension, tachycardia, and tachypnea may indicate sepsis. Redness, purulent drainage, and swelling of the site also may be observed in sepsis. Be sure to obtain a sample of any suspicious drainage for culturing and, upon removal of the catheter, culture the catheter tip.
- Use final filters on all TPN solutions to help eliminate bacteria and particulate matter and to prevent air emboli from entering the system.
- Educate the patient about self-care. Teach the patient to report any pain, redness, or swelling at the I.V. insertion site as well as any leakage along the I.V. tubing.
- Use a second I.V. line for administration of intermittent medications.
- Avoid administering medications and blood products via the I.V. line used for TPN to decrease the risk of contamination. Note that another port may be used when a triple-lumen catheter is used.

12
PEDIATRIC I.V. THERAPY

When providing intravenous (I.V.) therapy to a child, it is important to remember that the same complications that occur with adult I.V. therapy also can occur with pediatric I.V. therapy. Unfortunately, though, these problems tend to happen more quickly because children are smaller. Therefore, developing keen assessment skills and an ability to understand and relate to children is essential.

For many nurses, taking care of a child, especially one who is very sick and needs I.V. therapy, can be frightening and stressful. The parents of a sick child are also frightened and may express their fear as anxiety, timidness, or aggressiveness, further compounding a stressful situation.

When I.V. therapy is a part of a child's treatment, pain caused by catheter insertion is inevitable. The best analgesic in this situation is a combination of compassion for what the child is about to experience and constant explanation of the procedure to the child and parents. Be receptive to questions that anyone may have. Taking time to answer questions will decrease anxiety and set the mood for initiating an I.V. line in a calmer atmosphere.

Speak confidently and knowledgeably. Depending on the child's age, speak directly to the child. The parents may automatically assume responsibility for explaining what will occur. If this happens, remain quiet but stand by to answer questions. Then, introduce yourself to the child and begin the procedure.

Children are amazing; just when you think a child will fight, scream, and kick, he may simply cry louder than anyone thinks possible and manage to hold his arm still. Never assume that, because a child is only 4 years old, he is going to be difficult to hold. Take precautions and plan ahead. Take time to speak to the child, explaining that you need his help to do the best job you can. Promise you will do your best to give only one needle. Granted, this approach does not always work, but more times than not, the child will do his best to participate.

PREPARATION FOR INFUSION AND EQUIPMENT SELECTION

An I.V. setup for a child differs from an adult setup in that the flow rate may be minimal and the proper choice of tubing is important. The best choice for adequate control of a slow I.V. rate is microdrip tubing, and a mechanical monitoring device is highly recommended to deliver the minimal rate sometimes ordered for children. Its precise monitoring of the system will help prevent fluid overload.

Use extreme caution when using a pump to infuse I.V. fluid to a child. It takes very little fluid to cause serious infiltration in children because of their small size. Infiltrations occur, manifest, and become a serious problem very quickly. Therefore, hourly site evaluation is vital. Keep in mind that the pump does not detect such problems as phlebitis and early infiltrations.

If a monitoring device is unavailable, it is strongly recommended to use tubing with a volumetric chamber where small portions of the I.V. solutions can be added hourly. The chamber should have no more than 1 hour's worth of fluid at any given time to control the possibility of large volume overload if the clamping device is tampered with or fails.

The choice of equipment can aid in easier insertion and can prolong the life of the I.V. site. Choosing the smallest catheter to do the job will cause less I.V. trauma at the site and prolong the life of the infusion. Consider the tests and treatments the child will undergo, and be sure that the catheter gauge will be adequate in case special I.V. solutions or medications are required.

Children, especially infants, may have very limited venous access. A highly recommended practice is to check to see whether blood work has been ordered before starting the infusion. Keep in mind that, even though some laboratory specimens can be obtained via fingerstick, blood also can be obtained from the I.V. catheter. This will prevent numerous venipunctures and unnecessary trauma and allow for future access to an already limited number of veins.

When drawing blood from a catheter for laboratory tests, use a syringe that has at least a 6-cc capacity. Smaller syringes, such as 3-cc or tuberculin syringes, pull with too much pressure and can cause the vein to collapse. Too much pressure also can cause blood cells to hemolyze. Withdraw the plunger of the syringe slowly, taking about 1 to 1½ minutes to fill the syringe.

Drawing blood with too much pressure also may cause vein trauma, predisposing the vein to phlebitis. Remember, the innermost layer of vein is only one cell thick. Removing that delicate layer is very traumatic to the vein.

A major concern in starting an I.V. line in a child is keeping the child from moving. Papoose devices may be used if other people are unavailable to assist with the procedure. However, another person's assistance best helps with the taping, especially if the child is very young. Extra hands are always appreciated in pediatrics, no matter what the procedure.

Starting the I.V. line is the same with children as with adults (see Chapter 6, Performing the Procedures), but keep in mind that the sites available are limited. Veins in the hands, feet, scalp (usually only visible in infants), and antecubital areas usually are the only choices, and they must last the entire length of therapy.

When assessing the pediatric patient for venous access, consider the possibility of inserting a peripherally inserted central catheter (PICC) or midline catheter. However, one consideration is whether the child will tolerate the procedure, which is more involved than inserting a peripheral I.V. line. Other considerations include:

- What specific type of I.V. therapy has been ordered? Administration of total parenteral nutrition, administration of irritating medications, or I.V. therapy lasting 10 days or longer is a good reason for insertion of a catheter that accesses larger veins and has the potential to last longer.
- Will the child need to be sedated to perform the procedure, and will sedation compromise the child's condition? Light sedation and use of eutectic mixture of local anesthetics (EMLA) cream has proven very helpful in the success of PICC insertion for children.
- What is the child's activity level and the family's capacity to assist with caring for the catheter? Careful assessment of the most suitable catheter and catheter placement are important parts of vein preservation. PICC catheters greatly reduce the risk of chemical irritation and repeated venipuncture.

The tips offered in *Basic Procedures for Starting a Pediatric I.V. Line,* page 147, and *More Tips for Starting a Pediatric I.V. Line,* pages 148 to 150, are intended to assist nurses in preparing an I.V. infusion for a child.

MONITORING FOR COMPLICATIONS

Starting an I.V. line in a child is not the only difficulty in pediatric I.V. therapy. Once an I.V. line is established, the child must be monitored for complications (see Chapter 7, Complications). The most dangerous complication in children may be fluid overload. Because the body surface area of children varies greatly, the slightest change in the dosage or amount of fluid infused may severely alter the child's response to the infusate. To an infant, an additional 5 to 10 ml of fluid in 1 hour can cause fluid overload very rapidly, whereas it may not affect an adult at all.

On the same note, children become dehydrated faster than adults because they have a higher metabolic rate per unit of mass, so I.V. fluids become necessary to treat dehydration. Accurate fluid assessment is mandatory; strict monitoring of intake and output monitoring is essential in preventing overload and in achieving adequate hydration.

Because infants and children have a high metabolic rate, their water losses and maintenance requirements also are greater. All assessments for fluid loss should be based on the child's admission weight, body temperature, urine output, gastrointestinal (GI) losses (vomiting and diarrhea), skin turgor, and oral and ophthalmic secretions. These parameters plus insensible losses and stool consistency are guidelines for fluid replacement (see Chapter 1, Introduction to I.V. Therapy, for further details).

To determine necessary fluid maintenance, estimate the child's body weight before dehydration. Maintaining a child at this weight is more

(Text continues on page 151.)

BASIC PROCEDURES FOR STARTING A PEDIATRIC I.V. LINE

Action	Rationale
1. Assemble the necessary equipment (see Chapter 5, Selecting an I.V. Site, for details).	**1.** Having the equipment ready will save time and help decrease anxiety.
2. Prepare to obtain blood if necessary. Call laboratory personnel to receive blood, or assemble equipment for transfer of blood into the appropriate tubes.	**2.** This will eliminate the need for additional venipunctures. Extra hands also allow the nurse to focus on the I.V. site while others can help with the transfer of blood into the appropriate tubes.
3. Set up the necessary equipment to start the I.V. line.	**3.** Having tape torn and dressing equipment handy for quick securing of the catheter will prevent the possibility of losing the I.V. line as a result of patient movement.
4. Introduce yourself, stating your title, to the child and parents.	**4.** This helps both the child and parents feel secure and establishes your credibility.
5. Explain the procedure in a confident tone.	**5.** This indicates to the parents that the nurse who is about to insert an I.V. line in their child is knowledgeable and confident.
6. Answer any questions that the parents or child may have.	**6.** This helps alleviate fears of the unknown.
7. Do not overexplain or procrastinate.	**7.** Once a child knows that he or she will be receiving a needle, it is best to insert it as quickly as possible to prevent further anxieties.
8. Don gloves and start the I.V. procedure (see Chapter 6, Performing the Procedures, for details).	**8.** Gloves are necessary to prevent contamination.
9. Explain signs and symptoms of complications to the parents and child.	**9.** Educated parents and children (usually older children) often detect problems early.
10. Document the procedure; include date and time, gauge and type of cannula used, number of venipuncture attempts, patient's tolerance of procedure, and patient's or family's educational needs.	**10.** Proper documentation enables other staff members to know the capabilities of the I.V. site, inappropriate I.V. sites specific to the patient, and how often the site should be changed.

MORE TIPS FOR STARTING A PEDIATRIC I.V. LINE

● Elicit extra help, especially if the child is an infant. Remember that children have small arms and very small hands, making it difficult to find ample space for starting and taping the I.V. line. Another pair of hands may be necessary to prevent the catheter from accidentally dislodging once the vein is accessed.

● Try to start the I.V. line with the available help and apply the armboard only if necessary. If the board should become soiled with blood or solution, this moist area would provide a perfect medium for colonization of bacteria. Also, with a very active child, trying to change the board once the I.V. line has been established is risky. Furthermore, it may be necessary to move the limb around to access the vein.

● Perform the procedure somewhere other than the child's bed, such as in the treatment room. The child's bed should be used only for sleeping and playing. Starting an I.V. line there may cause a great deal of psychological trauma to a child.

● Ask the parents if they would prefer to remain in the room or step out. They may be helpful to the child and the nurse, if they are willing to hold the child. However, some children are more cooperative if family members are absent. Evaluate the situation carefully and suggest to the parents that their presence may be required or that the procedure may be easier without them present.

● Avoid using a scalp-vein needle (SVN) in children because children tend to pull at their dressings and the device can easily be dislodged. A dislodged SVN may stick the child in another place, presenting the chance of an infection or tissue damage elsewhere. Over-the-needle catheters are recommended in small children because they cannot cause addditional puncture once the stylet is removed.

● In small children, look for veins in the hands, antecubital areas, and feet. Note that the antecubital area is the best place to obtain a good blood return when blood samples are needed. Sometimes, obtaining blood from hand and foot veins is difficult because they are so small and collapse easily. Veins of the hands and feet are associated with an increased incidence of phlebitis because of their size and because they are difficult to secure. In a pinch, the antecubital vein is usually the easiest to access.

● Check your facility's policy on using scalp veins on infants. This can be tricky because it is difficult to establish the direction of blood flow. Some facilities prefer that this procedure be done by doctors and specially trained nurses, such as neonatal intensive care nurses and pediatric intensive care nurses.

● Keep in mind that small veins may collapse or spasm easily upon insertion, causing the blood return to cease. Wait 1 or 2 seconds to see if the return begins before considering the venipuncture unsuccessful. It even may be necessary to start the I.V. fluid dripping slowly to help dilate the vein and to ensure the device is properly placed. However, watch very closely for signs of infiltration, which indicates improper placement. *Note:* Never use vesicant or irritating solutions to check I.V. line placement — tissue damage may result.

● Try to keep the tape used to secure the catheter separate from the tape used to secure the limb to the armboard. When securing the I.V. site, tape the catheter to the arm. Never use the same piece of tape on the catheter hub that is used to secure the arm to the armboard. The child can work the arm, foot, or hand out of the tape, thus pulling the catheter out of the vein. (See the illustration in *Securing an I.V. Line in a Child's Hand.*)

Securing an I.V. in a child's hand

Apply the dressing to the site, then secure the padded armboard to the limb.

Do not secure the board with the same tape that secures the dressing.

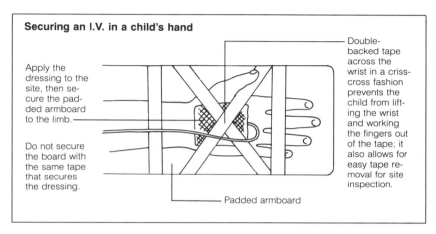

Double-backed tape across the wrist in a criss-cross fashion prevents the child from lifting the wrist and working the fingers out of the tape; it also allows for easy tape removal for site inspection.

Padded armboard

• When an I.V. line is inserted in the foot, taping usually is difficult. It sometimes helps to place an armboard on the side of the foot and tape a large amount of folded gauze to the board along the bottom of the foot. This will prevent foot movement. (See the illustration in *Securing an I.V. Line in a Child's Foot.*)

Securing an I.V. in a child's foot

Double-backed tape

Dressing is applied to I.V. site prior to criss-crossing at the ankle.

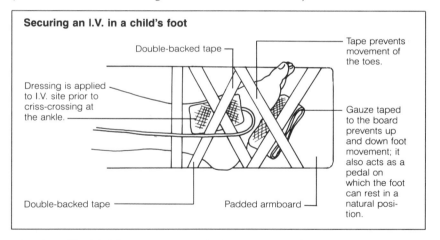

Tape prevents movement of the toes.

Gauze taped to the board prevents up and down foot movement; it also acts as a pedal on which the foot can rest in a natural position.

Double-backed tape

Padded armboard

• Another difficult I.V. line to tape is one in the small hand of a 1-week-old neonate. It is sometimes helpful to use a tongue depressor as an extension of the hand. It can be applied as an armboard. Folded gauze under the tubing will help to provide a surface to secure the line. The hardest part is ensuring that the fingers are flat on the tongue depressor so that the neonate will not be able to curl them and work them out of the tape. (See the illustration in *Securing an I.V. Line in a Neonate's Hand.*)

(continued)

MORE TIPS FOR STARTING A PEDIATRIC I.V. LINE *(continued)*

Securing an I.V. in a neonate's hand

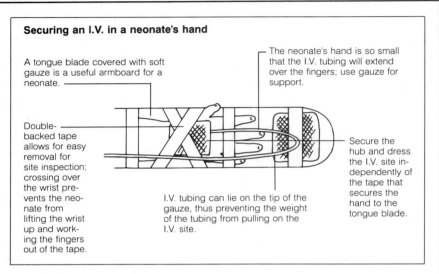

A tongue blade covered with soft gauze is a useful armboard for a neonate. ——

The neonate's hand is so small that the I.V. tubing will extend over the fingers; use gauze for support.

Double-backed tape allows for easy removal for site inspection; crossing over the wrist prevents the neonate from lifting the wrist up and working the fingers out of the tape.

I.V. tubing can lie on the tip of the gauze, thus preventing the weight of the tubing from pulling on the I.V. site.

Secure the hub and dress the I.V. site independently of the tape that secures the hand to the tongue blade.

• Explain the signs and symptoms of complications to the parents and child. They are the closest to the infusion at all times, so they can ensure that the line functions properly. Tell them to watch for swelling and redness at the site. Ask them to report anything that seems different or out of the ordinary to the nurse, including loose tape, beeping machines, and fluid drip cessation. This will help prevent problems and allow early detection of complications.

• Avoid completely covering the fingers and toes so that they may be assessed. Infected and gangrenous digits can result from poor circulation due to overtaping of I.V. sites.

• Explain to the parents that the tape may look tight on the child's "chubby" arm, but it is necessary to maintain security. Show the parents how to check for adequate circulation by squeezing the nailbeds and watching for blanching. The color of the fingers is also a good guide for adequate circulation.

• Perform hourly checks when a child has an I.V. line. Check for adequate circulation, signs of infiltration, and indicators of pain, such as squirming or crying when the vein is palpated. If a calm child cries when initiating I.V. medication, suspect that the child may be experiencing pain at the I.V. site.

• When securing the limb to an armboard, be sure that placement of the board allows for proper anatomical alignment. It is recommended that the board be placed after the site is accessed and the dressing is applied. Some prefer to place the board before inserting the catheter; although this practice is acceptible, the board may become soiled with blood and need to changed anyway.

• Use a soft roll of gauze, such as Kling, to help secure the site and prevent the child from playing with the I.V. site. This is acceptable as long as the site is visualized hourly and the fingertips and toes are accessible. Frequently, the gauze is not removed hourly, preventing thorough observation of the I.V. site.

important than maintaining the child at the present, dehydrated weight. Normal weight can be estimated by approximating weight loss as follows:

Mild dehydration = loss of 5% or less in body weight
Moderate dehydration = loss of 5% to 10% in body weight
Severe dehydration = loss of more than 15% in body weight
(near shock)

For example, a child weighing 10 kg is admitted to the hospital with a history of vomiting and diarrhea that has persisted for more than 24 hours. After careful assessment, the physician determines that the child is moderately dehydrated. In order to calculate the child's normal weight, consider the following:

Admission weight: 10 kg
Normal weight: X
Estimated body weight lost: 10%

Subtract the estimated weight loss (10%) from total body weight (100%) to obtain the dehydrated weight. In this case, 100% − 10% = 90%. If "X" equals the child's body weight before dehydration, then 9/10 X equals dehydrated weight (in this example, 10 kg). Therefore,

$$9/10 \text{ X} = 10 \text{ kg}$$
$$\text{X} = 100/9 \text{ kg}$$
$$\text{X} = 11.1 \text{ kg}$$

Thus, this child is estimated to have weighed approximately 11 kg before dehydration occurred. After this weight is obtained, daily fluid maintenance can be determined according to various charts and formulas designed for this purpose.

One formula that often is used follows:

100 ml/kg normal body weight for first 10 kg,
50 ml/kg of normal body weight for next 10 kg, and
20 ml/kg of normal body weight thereafter.

Total amount added together gives the amount of fluid required per day.

Here are some examples:
1. A child weighing 10 lb (4.5 kg) should receive 450 ml of fluid per day.
2. A child weighing 30 lb (14 kg) should receive 1,200 ml of fluid per day.
3. A child weighing 50 lb (23 kg) should receive 1,560 ml of fluid per day.

Another method for determining proper fluid replacement is the use of a body surface area nomogram (see *Using a Nomogram to Calculate Body Surface Area in Children*). By plotting the child's

USING A NOMOGRAM TO CALCULATE BODY SURFACE AREA IN CHILDREN

The following examples have been plotted to show how to correctly use a body surface area nomogram. The body surface area is determined by laying a straightedge on the child's height and weight and noting where the line intersects on the surface area scale in the center. The correct fluid replacement can be calculated using the formulas found on page 151.

Examples:

1. Child weighs 10 lb (4.5 kg) and is 22″ (56 cm) long. His body surface area equals approximately 0.28 m² His fluid replacement should be approximately 420 ml/day.

2. Child weighs 30 lb (14 kg) and is 37″ (94 cm) tall. Her body surface area equals approximately 0.62 m² Her fluid replacement should be approximately 930 ml/day.

3. Child weighs 50 lb (23 kg) and is 48″ (122 cm) tall. His body surface area equals approximately 0.9 m² His fluid replacement should be approximately 1,350 ml/day.

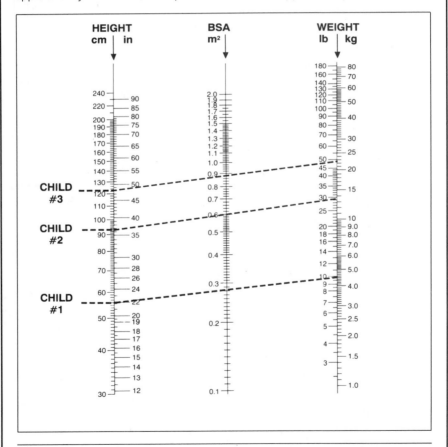

Adapted with permission from Behrman, et. al. *Nelson Textbook of Pediatrics*, 14th edition. W.B. Saunders Co.: Philadelphia, 1992.

weight in kilograms and height in centimeters, one can obtain the body surface area in square meters by drawing a line from each point and intersecting a point on the center graph of a chart. This value is then used to calculate the amount of fluid to be replaced in 24 hours, using the following formula: 1,500 ml/m².

SPECIAL CONSIDERATIONS
In emergencies, a specially prepared crash cart is used for children. Code situations may call for an immediate I.V. line, used to provide venous access so that lifesaving medications can be given via I.V. push or infusion.

Because of the difference in the dosages of the medications listed, steps must be taken to avoid the possibility of errors. The smallest alteration in the child's dosage of a medication can cause a dramatic difference in the patient's expected response.

It is a wise, timesaving idea to prepare, on admission, a list of emergency drugs and dosages based on weight for each child, and to display it at the bedside. This is especially helpful in pediatric intensive care units and emergency departments, where arrest situations are most likely to occur. Figuring out the dosage of each medication on admission will reduce errors that a code situation could cause. Computer programs are available to calculate the emergency drug dosages according to the child's weight. The computer calculates the dosages and prints a copy for the child's chart or for posting at the child's bedside.

I.V. therapy in children presents many challenges. Anxious, frightened parents may cause difficulties in their child's treatment; patience and understanding help. Explain as much as possible to the child and parents before beginning any kind of treatment, so they know what to expect. It might be helpful to construct a letter to give to parents, so that they may prepare their child for venipuncture (see *Sample Letter to Parents,* page 154).

Children are special and deserve special attention and assistance. Always do your best to make a frightening experience less traumatic for these special young people. Talk to them soothingly and remember to explain all procedures to them, but do not allow them to procrastinate. Remember, compassion and constant explanation are the best analgesics for helping a child through I.V. insertion. Also, do it and get it over with as quickly and as confidently as possible.

SAMPLE LETTER TO PARENTS

Dear Parent:

The doctor has ordered intravenous (I.V.) therapy for your child. I.V. therapy is used for many reasons. For example, if your child suffers vomiting or diarrhea or a high fever, he or she will need I.V. therapy to replace body fluids.

Although most medications can be given by mouth or by injection, they are not as fast-acting or as effective as ones given through the veins. By giving medications intravenously, your child will receive only one needle, whereas with injections, your child may receive a needle every few hours for several days. Therefore, I.V. therapy is much less traumatic.

You may be asked to leave the room or to allow the nurse to take your child to a treatment room to perform the procedure. The nurse is experienced in inserting I.V. lines and will take good care of your child. If you are to remain with your child during the procedure, you can help by keeping your child from moving so that the nurse can successfully insert the needle on the first attempt.

Even under the best circumstances, a suitable vein may be difficult to find with one needlestick. Sometimes two or more needlesticks are necessary. No matter how experienced the nurse is at venipuncture, one attempt cannot be guaranteed. So please do not promise your child that there will be only one. It will only frighten your child if the first one is not successful.

The nurse will choose the vein and insert the I.V. line. The metal needle inside the plastic tube (catheter) will be taken out and the tube will remain in the vein. It will be taped in place, and an armboard will be used to secure the I.V. line and stabilize the limb. When the catheter is in position, your child will experience no pain. However, if pain does occur, be sure to tell the nurse. Also, please inform the nurse of any swelling, redness, or loose tape around the I.V. site. This will help the nurse to act on any problems as early as possible.

When the I.V. line is started, blood may be obtained for laboratory studies to prevent your child from receiving excessive needlesticks. However, it is not always possible to get the necessary amount from a child's small, delicate veins. If an adequate amount of blood cannot be obtained, the phlebotomist will have to obtain a specimen from another vein or by fingerstick, depending on which test is being done.

When the I.V. line is taped in place, please remind your child not to touch or pick at the tape. This could loosen the I.V. line or dislodge the catheter, and another venipuncture may be needed. Soft restraints may be used if your child cannot leave the I.V. line alone.

We understand that you are not with your child every minute, but when you are here, your assistance is important and greatly appreciated. The nurses will observe the I.V. line often, even throughout the night.

If you have any questions, please feel free to ask them. Thank you for taking the time to read this letter and for helping us prepare your child for I.V. therapy. It will benefit us all, especially our little patient.

Your I.V. Nurses

APPENDIX A:
NURSING PLANS OF CARE

These nursing plans of care are designed for any patient receiving I.V. therapy, including children. Review and adapt this information to provide each patient with optimal, safe intravenous (I.V.) therapy.

Nursing diagnosis	Nursing intervention	Rationale
GENERAL I.V. THERAPY		
Anxiety related to I.V. therapy and disease process *Patient outcome:* Patient will verbalize a decrease in anxiety level.	**1.** Assess the patient's and family's regular coping mechanisms.	**1.** Familiar coping mechanisms can be used to lower anxiety.
	2. Provide realistic, positive reassurance; also answer the patient's questions.	**2.** Positive, realistic reassurance and answers help develop positive rapport and trust with the patient.
	3. Involve the patient's family in care.	**3.** Using existing support systems, such as parents or friends, increases the patient's comfort level.
	4. Provide diversionary activities, especially for children.	**4.** This helps reduce anxiety about illness and I.V. therapy and provides another method of coping.
	5. Prepare the patient for any intervention before initiating the activity.	**5.** Abrupt initiation of any intervention can decrease receptiveness, rapport, and compliance by increasing anxiety.
	6. Avoid prolonging the procedure.	**6.** Prolonging the procedure allows time for anxiety to increase.
Sleep pattern disturbance related to I.V. therapy and underlying disease *Patient outcome:* The patient will sleep comfortably at night with minimal disruptions.	**1.** Assess the patient's usual sleep patterns. (Ask the parents to supply this information for a child.)	**1.** This may help identify problems with regular sleeping patterns; for instance, napping during day may affect the patient's ability to sleep at night.
	2. Suggest diversionary activities during the day for stimulation.	**2.** Diversionary activities will stimulate the patient during the day so that he or she will be tired at night.
	3. Discuss the patient's feelings about the disease, I.V. therapy medications, and I.V. equipment.	**3.** Anxiety about the disease or malfunction of equipment delivering medication can cause sleep disturbances.
	4. Instruct the patient about the safe use and reliability of I.V. equipment. Reassure the patient that the part of the I.V. that remains in the vein is plastic, not metal (unless scalp-vein needle is used). Show the patient an I.V. line without a needle.	**4.** Anxiety over being "stabbed" with a needle, having the needle break while in the vein, or having metal in the arm can cause sleep disturbances.

Nursing diagnosis	Nursing intervention	Rationale
GENERAL I.V. THERAPY		
Sleep pattern disturbance related to I.V. therapy and underlying disease *(continued)*	**5.** Explain that the method used to taping an I.V. line will help keep it from falling out.	**5.** Anxiety about the catheter falling out and the possible need to repeat procedure can cause sleep disturbances.
	6. Show the patient the correct procedure for using the call button to contact the nurse. Repeat your name before leaving the patient and family.	**6.** Proper instruction and reassurance builds confidence and decreases anxiety, thereby reducing the chance of sleep disturbances.
Body image disturbance related to I.V. therapy and underlying disease *Patient outcome:* The patient will demonstrate a positive body-image; if a child, the patient will demonstrate appropriate social developmental characteristics.	**1.** Assess the patient for psychosocial problems or problems with or changes in activities of daily living (ADLs). Specifically, assess for: ● altered rapport with family and friends ● changes in routine ADLs ● interference from the I.V. line that might disrupt range of motion or other daily activities ● uneasiness over having a foreign object in the body ● fear of catheter dislocation ● fear of others' reaction to the I.V. line.	**1.** Identifying changes in lifestyle and psychosocial problems facilitates an understanding of the patient's feelings and determines the need for intervention. Encourage the patient and family to verbalize feelings regarding the disease and therapy. In the case of a child, this may entail the use of play therapy (such as a doll with an I.V. connected to it).
	2. Answer the patient's and family's questions about the underlying disease and I.V. therapy as simply as possible.	**2.** Knowing more about the situation will help the patient to feel less alienated and more comforted. Verbalizing feelings and concerns also enables the patient to recognize problems and develop effective coping methods.
	3. Encourage the physician to clearly explain the disease and to answer the patient and family's questions.	**3.** This will provide a better understanding and facilitate team communication.
Pain related to I.V. insertion, limited positioning, adverse drug effects, and underlying disease *Patient outcome:* The patient will not complain of discomfort and will show no signs of pain.	**1.** Assess the patient for signs of pain or discomfort, including the location, duration, and quality of pain and any precipitating factors. Also assess for any pain or discomfort related to: ● the I.V. catheter's position, patency, and site ● the underlying disease ● drug adverse reactions ● I.V. site and venous pathway.	**1.** A malpositioned catheter can limit range of motion and cause pain; phlebitis and infection can stimulate the pain response; and the disease itself can produce pain. Therefore, determining the cause of pain will affect appropriate treatment.

Nursing diagnosis	Nursing intervention	Rationale

GENERAL I.V. THERAPY

Nursing diagnosis	Nursing intervention	Rationale
Pain related to I.V. insertion, limited positioning, adverse drug effects, and underlying disease *(continued)*	**2.** Document any complaints of pain. Also, notify the physician if the pain or discomfort is severe or interferes with ADLs; obtain orders for appropriate treatment, and evaluate the patient's response.	**2.** Documentation and proper physician notification acknowledges the reality of the pain and allows for prompt pain relief.
	3. Instruct the patient and family to inform the nurse and physician about any discomfort. Also demonstrate proper I.V. catheter positioning to patient and family.	**3.** Patient and family education promotes compliance and minimizes the risk of problems.
	4. Instruct the patient and family about adverse drug effects, and advise them to report them to the nurse or physician. Also inform them about any medication or dosage changes.	**4.** The patient can experience adverse effects to any medication. Adverse effects (such as gastrointestinal [GI] upset and shortness of breath) can cause discomfort and pain. Proper instruction promotes communication of the problem so that prompt intervention can occur; the physician must be made aware of adverse effects in order to prescribe a different medication or a change in the medication's dosage.
	5. Answer the patient's questions, and provide realistic, positive reassurance.	**5.** Answering questions honestly alleviates anxiety, promotes the comfort, and improves compliance.
Altered skin integrity related to I.V. puncture site *Patient outcomes:* — The patient will be free of infection at the I.V. site, and the site will heal properly after discontinuance of therapy. — The patient will be free of signs of phlebitis during I.V. therapy. — The patient will be free of complications of infiltration during the course of I.V. therapy.	**1.** Assess the I.V. site for signs of redness, irritation, or drainage. Check the limb for pain, swelling, blanching, temperature changes, and presence of a cordlike vein; also compare both arms for evidence of infiltration and systemic edema. Make sure that tape is not wrapped too tightly around the I.V. site (this is especially important for children). **2.** Change the I.V. site every 72 hours. Change the I.V. site dressing daily and as ordered, and maintain aseptic technique.	**1.** A break in the skin (such as at a puncture site) provides an excellent port of entry for microbes. Both arms should be compared to verify bilateral edema or infiltration. Tape placed too tightly can obstruct the fluid flow, making a child's baby fat look like an infiltrate. **2.** Aseptic technique and frequent assessment lowers incidence of phlebitis. Leaving peripheral catheters in place longer than 72 hours increases the risk of phlebitis; improper site care provides a foundation for bacterial growth.

Nursing diagnosis	Nursing intervention	Rationale

GENERAL I.V. THERAPY

Nursing diagnosis	Nursing intervention	Rationale
Altered skin integrity related to I.V. puncture sites *(continued)*	**3.** Instruct the patient and family to notify the nurse if they notice signs and symptoms of infection or if the dressing becomes wet.	**3.** Notifying the nurse will ensure prompt infection control measures.
	4. Take necessary measures to decrease movement of the catheter, including taping the I.V. line securely and using an armboard to prevent movement of limb and catheter.	**4.** Securing the I.V. prevents I.V. movement and further skin disruption or vein damage.
	5. Assess the I.V. line for patency before administering any fluid or medication.	**5.** Ensuring I.V. patency is essential prior to administering any fluid or medication to prevent complications, including infection.
Altered tissue perfusion related to emboli *Patient outcome:* The patient will be free of any signs or symptoms of decreased circulation.	**1.** Assess for signs and symptoms of embolic episodes, including decreased circulation to an extremity, pain, cyanosis, cool skin, sudden onset of shortness of breath or respiratory difficulty, changes in mental status (decreased sensorium, altered affect), changes in muscle tone, decreased use of extremity, and changes in speech.	**1.** Thorough assessment is necessary to determine the nature of embolic episodes and appropriate treatment.
	2. Teach the patient and family to recognize and report signs and symptoms of embolism.	**2.** Early recognition will ensure prompt intervention.
	3. Maintain patency of the I.V. line by using the correct flush procedure.	**3.** Flushing the line correctly will minimize clot formation at the tip of the catheter.
	4. Avoid forcing fluid through the catheter. If resistance is met, try to withdraw blood and establish a flow. If unable to do this, discontinue I.V. line.	**4.** Forcing fluid through the catheter may introduce a thrombus into the circulatory system, causing an embolic episode.
Risk for infection related to I.V. therapy *Patient outcome:* The patient will be free of any complications of infection during the course of I.V. therapy.	**1.** Assess the I.V. site daily, and teach the patient and family to recognize and report signs and symptoms of infection, including localized pain, redness, inflammation, drainage, changes in vital signs, and elevated temperature. If signs of	**1.** If infection occurs, early recognition of signs and symptoms aids in prompt treatment.

Nursing diagnosis	Nursing intervention	Rationale

GENERAL I.V. THERAPY

Nursing diagnosis	Nursing intervention	Rationale
Risk for infection related to I.V. therapy *(continued)*	infection occur, discontinue the I.V., remove the catheter, call the physician, culture the catheter tip, and document the incident in the patient's chart.	
	2. Assess for signs and symptoms of sepsis, including lethargy, malaise, loss of appetite, diaphoresis, elevated temperature, neurologic changes, and seizures.	**2.** Early detection of sepsis ensures prompt treatment.
	3. Keep the I.V. dressing clean and secure; change according to institutional policy. Change the peripheral I.V. cannula at least every 72 hours. Change the I.V. tubing according to institutional policy; usually, this is every 72 hours unless the tubing is connected to a central I.V. line or being used to administer total parenteral nutrition (TPN). For central I.V. lines and TPN lines, the tubing should be changed every 24 hours. I.V. lines used to administer medications that tend to form precipitates (such as Dilantin) require a tubing change with each dose.	**3.** Proper changing methods and maintaining asepsis help to minimize the risk of infection.
	4. Change the dressing if it becomes wet or soiled. Keep the I.V. site clean of other drainage, such as from a wound or tracheostoma.	**4.** Wet or soiled tape provides an excellent medium for bacterial growth. Drainage should be kept away from any opening in the skin to prevent contamination.
Fluid volume deficit or excess related to I.V. therapy *Patient outcome:* The patient will exhibit signs of fluid balance.	**1.** Assess the patient's intake and output for signs of overhydration or dehydration, as applicable. Teach the patient and family to accurately obtain fluid intake and output measurements and when to notify the nurse of imbalances.	**1.** Closely monitored intake and output can reduce the chance of fluid overload or fluid deficit.

Nursing diagnosis	Nursing intervention	Rationale

GENERAL I.V. THERAPY

Nursing diagnosis	Nursing intervention	Rationale
Fluid volume deficit or excess related to I.V. therapy *(continued)*	● When measuring intake, include all fluids given, such as I.V. fluids, nasogastric (NG) tube feedings, blood and blood by-products, and hemodynamic monitoring flushes. ● When measuring output, include all fluids excreted, such as urine, diarrhea, GI suctioning, and drainage from wounds.	
	2. Check the patient's weight daily.	**2.** An increase in weight reflects a gain of fluid (a 1-lb weight gain equals a fluid gain of 2 liters). Similarly, a decrease in weight reflects a loss of fluid (a 1-lb weight loss equals a fluid loss of 2 liters).
	3. Monitor the patient's vital signs for any changes; assess for crackles, shortness of breath, chest pain, extra heart sounds, neck vein distention, altered point of maximum impulse (PMI), and edema.	**3.** Fluid overload can be detected by changes in vital signs.
	4. Assess for orthostatic hypotension, thirst, flattened neck veins, dry mucous membranes, and diminished skin turgor.	**4.** These signs indicate fluid volume deficit and require treatment.
	5. Closely monitor the intake and output of all pediatric patients.	**5.** Small variations in the amount of fluid can have disastrous effects in a child.

MEDICATION ADMINISTRATION

Nursing diagnosis	Nursing intervention	Rationale
Knowledge deficit related to medication therapy *Patient outcome:* The patient and family will verbalize an understanding of all aspects of the medication therapy regimen.	**1.** Assess the patient's and family's initial understanding.	**1.** This establishes a baseline of knowledge from which to work.
	2. Instruct the patient and family about the medication's dosage, therapeutic effect, adverse effects, drug interactions, and any other special instructions or precautions.	**2.** Such knowledge promotes confidence about the treatment as well as confidence in the staff and increases the likelihood that they will comply with the medication regimen.
	3. Teach the patient and family the signs and symptoms of adverse reactions and the importance of notifying the physician as soon as any occur.	**3.** This increases the likelihood of compliance and ensures prompt intervention should adverse effects occur.

Nursing diagnosis	Nursing intervention	Rationale

TOTAL PARENTERAL NUTRITION

Knowledge deficit related to the purpose, function, and administration of total parenteral nutrition (TPN) *Patient outcome:* The patient and family will verbalize an understanding of the reasons for TPN and how to administer it properly.	**1.** Assess the patient's and family's understanding of TPN as related to the underlying disease and the therapy's purpose, function, administration, and possible complications.	**1.** This establishes a baseline from which to work and helps the nurse develop an appropriate teaching plan.
	2. Ask the patient and family to describe in their own terms the TPN procedure and necessary equipment.	**2.** Identifying misconceptions and gaining familiarity with the patient's terminology will facilitate teaching and learning.
	3. Correct any misconceptions about the definition, purpose, administration, and associated complications of TPN, using terms the patient and family can understand.	**3.** Providing correct information in understandable terms will enhance compliance and promote confidence in the therapy and staff.
	4. Teach the patient and family to recognize signs and symptoms of complications and the importance of reporting them immediately to the physician. Provide specific information regarding hyperglycemia, hypoglycemia, sepsis, embolism, and altered GI function (such as anorexia and bowel changes).	**4.** Understanding the possible complications of therapy will ensure quick detection and early intervention.

CHEMOTHERAPY

Risk for impaired skin integrity related to chemotherapy *Patient outcome:* The patient will have no skin problems or complication resulting from extravasation.	**1.** Before initiating therapy, obtain specific guidelines from the physician regarding the proper extravasation procedure or antidote for the chemotherapeutic agent to be infused.	**1.** Following the proper procedure or using the prescribed antidote can reduce the agent's caustic effects and the severity of extravasation if treated promptly.
	2. Be aware of safety precautions while preparing and administering a vesicant, including the need to wear gloves and to observe for leakage at connection sites.	**2.** Using proper safety precautions minimizes the risk of skin damage during preparation and administration.
	3. Assess the I.V. site for signs of redness, swelling, and pain. If any of these signs are evident, immediately: • check to ensure that the device is secure and patent • remove the dressing	**3.** These signs indicate that the I.V. line is not patent. If medication is infused, extravasation can result, causing irreversible damage to underlying tendons and neuromuscular structures with functional joint impairment.

Nursing diagnosis	Nursing intervention	Rationale

CHEMOTHERAPY

Nursing diagnosis	Nursing intervention	Rationale
Risk for impaired skin integrity related to chemotherapy *(continued)*	• administer dextrose 5% in water (D₅W) as a free-flow infusion, flush with normal saline solution to check patency of cannula, and observe for infiltration. • check the flow rate (stop the flow immediately and call the physician if swelling is noted) • restart the I.V. line at another location, preferably in the other limb.	
	4. Infuse medication, as ordered, in 1-ml increments with intermittent D₅W or normal saline solution push. Check frequently for blood return and continually assess the site while infusing medication.	**4.** Monitoring blood return and the I.V. site ensures proper placement, which reduces the risk of extravasation and minimizes complications.
	5. Be aware of which medications are vesicants; these include dactinomycin (actinomycin D), daunorubicin, mitomycin, and vincristine. Tell the patient and family to report any burning, pain, or discomfort during the infusion.	**5.** One of the first signs of infiltration of a vesicant solution is burning and pain; early detection allows for prompt treatment.
Altered nutrition: less than body requirements related to the underlying disease, anorexia, nausea, and vomiting *Patient outcome:* The patient will maintain optimal nutritional status and will have minimal nausea and vomiting.	**1.** Assess the patient's regular eating and bowel habits, and identify any changes from the normal pattern.	**1.** This establishes a baseline and allows the nurse to act promptly to prevent malnutrition, dehydration, and electrolyte imbalance.
	2. Explain to the patient the effects of the underlying disease (if these have not already been openly discussed with physician) and the effects of chemotherapeutic agents on the GI system.	**2.** Awareness of the potential adverse reactions will help the patient to deal with the disturbances.
	3. Obtain a physician's order to premedicate the patient with antiemetics and sedatives.	**3.** Prophylactic antiemetics and sedatives can decrease the nausea and vomiting and indirectly increase the appetite of a patient undergoing chemotherapy.
	4. Instruct the patient on the proper use of antiemetics (administering every 4 hours with chemotherapy is known to produce nausea and vomiting).	**4.** To achieve a therapeutic effect, antiemetics should be administered before starting chemotherapy and at regular intervals as prescribed.

Nursing diagnosis	Nursing intervention	Rationale

CHEMOTHERAPY

Nursing diagnosis	Nursing intervention	Rationale
Risk for infection related to suppression of the immune response and bone marrow function *Patient outcome:* The patient will be free of signs and symptoms of depressed bone marrow function (stomatitis and bleeding) and infection.	**1.** Assess laboratory values, including complete blood count with differential, before and after treatment. **2.** Teach the patient and family preventive measures to decrease the risk of stomatitis, infection, and bleeding. **3.** Instruct the patient how to treat stomatitis, infection, and bleeding.	**1.** Changes in the bone marrow and immune system function from the immunosuppressant effects of chemotherapy can be determined by laboratory values. **2.** Preventive measures can reduce incidence and severity of adverse effects of chemotherapy. **3.** Adequate instruction promotes compliance and helps minimize the discomfort associated with these effects.
Body image disturbance related to alopecia associated with chemotherapy *Patient outcome:* The patient will maintain optimal body image and verbalize concerns.	**1.** When teaching about chemotherapy, inform the patient about the possibility of alopecia. Assess the patient's and family's normal coping mechanisms. **2.** Allow the patient and family to verbalize feelings, and provide emotional support. **3.** Assess for signs of alopecia. If present, suggest wearing hair pieces, scarves, and hats, as appropriate. **4.** Provide information on how to obtain financial assistance to obtain hairpieces, if necessary.	**1.** Assessment provides a baseline from which to proceed. Preparing the patient and family for the possibility of alopecia will allow them to mobilize resources to decrease stress. Relying on the patient's and family's existing coping mechanisms, if appropriate, helps decrease anxiety. **2.** Verbalization can reduce stress, decrease anxiety, and alleviate fear of the unknown. **3.** Such devices as hair pieces and scarves help minimize the body image effects of alopecia. **4.** The patient may desire a hairpiece but have insufficient funds to purchase one. Financial assistance can provide the patient with some sense of control.
Knowledge deficit related to complications of chemotherapy, including extravasation, alopecia, GI disturbances, stomatitis, infection, and bleeding *Patient outcome:* The patient will verbalize accurate information about possible complications and how to prevent and treat them.	**1.** Assess the patient's and family's understanding of the possible complications. **2.** Develop a teaching plan that effectively addresses the possible complications and their prevention and treatment.	**1.** Assessment provides a baseline from which to develop an appropriate teaching plan. **2.** Instructing the patient and family about the possibility of complications and specific ways to prevent and treat them will help decrease the incidence and severity of complications during therapy.

APPENDIX B: CONTINUOUS QUALITY IMPROVEMENT AND I.V. THERAPY

An important focus of health care for the 1990s is continuous quality improvement (CQI). Previously referred to as total quality management (TQM) and total quality improvement (TQI), CQI involves the collection, organization, and reporting of data using statistical analyses. According to the Intravenous Nurses Society (INS), statistical data reflective of CQI should be compiled, reviewed, and evaluated regularly to quantify and qualify outcomes of intravenous (I.V.) therapy.

A worksheet on which to collect data, record trends, evaluate products, and document daily I.V. care is a helpful tool for tracking CQI (see the sample worksheet on page 166). Each facility should develop its own worksheet and establish guidelines for collecting and recording data to make documentation easier and to ensure consistency among staff. The use of standard definitions and abbreviations that are easy to memorize simplifies the documentation procedure and helps to ensure compliance.

All I.V. catheters are removed for a particular reason; that reason should be documented and tracked carefully to determine where problems lie. Some examples of standard definitions and abbreviations that may be used on a worksheet are listed below:

- Protocol restart (PR) = Changing of an I.V. site that is healthy (without signs and symptoms of complications) simply because it has been in the same location for 72 hours (or 48 hours, depending on the facility's protocol)
- Phlebitis (P) = Redness of the I.V. site
- Infiltration (I) = Swelling at the I.V. site
- Clotting [or clogging] (C) = Obstruction of fluid drip in the I.V. line and/or inability to flush the I.V. cannula
- Leaking (L) = Blood or I.V. fluid leaking at the I.V. site
- Hurt (H) = Patient's complaint of discomfort although the I.V. site is healthy (could lead to phlebitis)
- Discontinued (DC) = Removal of any patent catheter from a healthy I.V. site prior to the established protocol (every 72 or 48 hours, depending on the facility)
- Other (O) = Any unidentifiable problem or problem not listed on the worksheet (such as accidental dislodging of catheter and patient's pulling and removal of catheter)

One staff member should be responsible for tallying all of the daily statistics at the end of the month and reporting the information. All of the members of the data collection team should be evaluated for the consistency of the data they collect, as this will lead to more consistent reporting.

The final report should reflect the total number of I.V. catheter removals for the month, broken down according to problem areas and stated in the form of percentages. For example, a final report might indicate the following information:

PR (protocol restarts) = 85% of all removals
P (phlebitis) = 4% of all removals
I (infiltration) = 2% of all removals
... and so on.

Plotting the percentages on a graph will enable your facility to track trends. After a few months, it will become evident which specific areas of I.V. therapy are especially problematic for your facility or individual unit. However, keep in mind that, regardless of which information is reported, you need to take into account certain variables. For instance, you need to consider the general age of the patients treated in your facility. The aging process has an obvious effect on veins and skin; therefore, age will be reflected in the statistics.

INS has established a standard for only phlebitis, which is less than 5% of all I.V. restarts. All other standards are set according to each facility's practices and patient population. Suggested goals for other reportable statistics are listed below:

● Protocol restarts should be the largest percentage of removals (the higher, the better), indicating that the care provided was adequate to keep the I.V. sites healthy for the facility's limit.

● Phlebitis should be below 5%, as established by INS guidelines, indicating that I.V. sites were inserted with minimal trauma and secured well to prevent vein trauma resulting from cannula manipulation. The quality of the catheter used also will be reflected here (the percentage will be higher if the cannula is known to cause peelback, resulting in endothelial lesions). The gauge that is most commonly used will also be reflected here; for example, surgical units, where large-gauge catheters are commonly used, may have a higher phlebitis rate. Bacterial phlebitis (reported by some infection control departments) should be eliminated or reduced to a minimum when an I.V. team starts the lines.

● Infiltrations are a little more complicated; one research report suggests that 25% of patients receiving I.V. therapy will experience infiltration. Many factors contribute to a high infiltration rate (for example, age of patients, skin [and vein] elasticity, length of therapy, use of pumps, skill level of nurses, available nursing time for attending to I.V. sites, security of I.V. site and cannula, and use of armboards). It often takes a few months of collected data (sometimes 6 months' worth) before any changes are made and to set a standard for the facility. However, once the common percentage is found, the facility should begin working immediately to decrease it. Generally, the older the population involved, the higher the average percentage will be. Also, when pumps are used for peripheral infusions and set on a high-pressure setting, the risk of infiltration tends to increase.

- Discontinued I.V. catheters also represent patent, healthy I.V. sites, so this percentage should be as high as possible.
- Clotted (or occluded) I.V. catheters are a common problem and require close watching. Frequently, a facility will see a correlation between the rise and fall of plotted phlebitis rates and clotted rates. If the rates are compared on a graph, some common peaks may be seen. It is suspected that proper catheter flushing will decrease the incidence of clotted I.V. lines, thereby decreasing irritation of the

CONTINUOUS QUALITY IMPROVEMENT

MONTH: _____ UNIT: _____

DATE	1	2	3	4	5	6	7	8	9	10	11	12	13	14	
CENSUS															
TOTAL STARTS															
PROTOCOL RESTART (PR)															
PHLEBITIS (P)															
HURT (H)															
INFILTRATION (I)															
CLOTTED (C)															
LEAKING (L)															
DISCONTIN-UED (DC)															
OTHER (O)															

I.V. TRACK	CENSUS	TOTAL STARTS	PR	P
MONTHLY TOTAL				
PERCENTAGE				

delicate vein walls. If the irritation decreases, the incidence of phlebitis is likely to decrease as well.

Because quality, consistent I.V. care is the goal, the entire I.V. team should look closely at the CQI monthly statistics and take the necessary steps to improve I.V. care, including providing in-service education to correct developing trends. It can be especially rewarding for nurses to see the numbers change in response to their hard work.

SHIFT: _____

	15	16	17	18	19	20	21	22	23	24	25	26	27	28	29	30	31

	H	I	C	L	DC	O

APPENDIX C:
TROUBLESHOOTING I.V. PROBLEMS

The following questions are representative of some of the most common problems nurses encounter when providing I.V. therapy. Read each question carefully, and answer as if you were caring for the patient yourself.

---

1. *The patient's arm looks healthy, without signs or symptoms of infiltration or phlebitis. The I.V. line runs well with the infusion device, but the machine "beeps" frequently. What is the problem?*

ANSWER: If the patient shows no signs of pain or complications and the I.V. line appears to be patent, secure, and running well, explore the following possibilities:
- Check to see whether the machine is plugged in and whether the battery is dead.
- Note whether the tubing's drip chamber is filled properly. (The drip chamber should be filled according to manufacturer's recommendation.)
- If your machine is a newer model, check to see whether the display panel identifies the reason for the beeping. (Most machines now are computerized and identify the reason for alarms sounding.)
- Check the manufacturer's handbook for troubleshooting tips if the machine is causing the problem. (The problem must be with the machine if the I.V. fluid runs well.)

---

2. *The I.V. site is clean and without complications. However, blood is dripping from somewhere. What is the problem?*

ANSWER: The problem actually depends on where the blood is dripping from. Check all connections; the cannula hub and tubing connection may have come apart. Also, if the I.V. fluid is in a bottle and a vented set is not used, a vaccum will be created in the system and blood may be pulled into the tubing.

---

3. *The patient appears to have edema in only one limb. The hand in which the I.V. line is placed is swollen and cool to the touch. The blood return is diluted. What is the problem?*

ANSWER: The I.V. line has become infiltrated, despite the presence of a blood return. The I.V. line should be discontinued and restarted above the infiltrated area or in the other limb. Warm compresses should be applied to the swollen area, and the extremity should be elevated on a pillow to promote circulation. (If chemotherapeutic agents, phenytoin, or dopamine caused the infiltration, you may need to apply ice; however, consult the physician and check your facilitiy's policy.)

4. *There are no signs of complications at the I.V. site. However, the tubing has come apart at the connection. The I.V. line does not run on the infusion device, but it runs for a short time on the pump. What is the problem?*

ANSWER: The I.V. line probably is clotted. The pump will build up pressure in the tubing, causing separation in an area between the pump and catheter if the resistance is less than the resistance of a clot. An I.V. line may drip for a short time when it is clotted. If a piggyback is hanging with an open clamp, the I.V. line will drip; however, instead of infusing into the patient, it will go to an area of "lesser" resistance — in this case, back up into the piggyback bag.

5. *The patient has an I.V. line in the forearm. The area around the I.V. site is generally red, painful to the touch, and swollen. What is the problem?*

ANSWER: The problem probably is a chemical irritation. Because phlebitis usually does not present with swelling, the I.V. line probably became infiltrated and the chemicals of the solution entered the tissue, causing a generalized redness. Elevate the limb and use ice or a warm compress, depending on the solution being infused, to soothe any discomfort and promote circulation.

6. *An I.V. catheter running by gravity with an open clamp drips only occasionally. The site has no signs of infiltration or phlebitis. What is the problem?*

ANSWER: The I.V. cannula needs to be repositioned. The tip of the cannula may be touching the wall of the vein or a valve, causing the I.V. line to stop dripping. A good way to check this is to carefully undress the I.V. line and slightly withdraw the cannula to see if a steady flow can be obtained. Observe the site for signs of infiltration. Then, resecure the I.V. in a better position.

7. *The patient has an I.V. line in the antecubital fossa. The insertion site is leaking. What is the problem?*

ANSWER: If blood is leaking from the site, the movement of the cannula may have torn the skin or expanded the vein opening, causing bleeding at the site. If clear I.V. solution is leaking, then the cannula is probably bent and cracked at the bend. Look for signs of local swelling at the site caused by I.V. solution leaking out of the cracked cannula under the skin. In both instances, the line should be discontinued very carefully to prevent cannula breakage and restarted in a more comfortable area.

8. *An extremely ill patient has an I.V. site that is swollen, but the solution is infusing well. She has extremely limited sites for restarting the I.V. line. There is a slight, diluted blood return. Should this line be left in until a better site is obtained?*

ANSWER: No! If the site is swollen, it probably is infiltrated; therefore, the solution is pooling under the skin. All of the solution is not going through the vein. One drop of a vesicant or irritating solution can cause major irritation or tissue damage. No solution should be allowed to collect in one spot. If the area is swollen, discontinue the line. The only exception to this is for an extremely edematous patient when infiltration is not suspected. In this particular case, both arms probably are swollen; if so, elevate the arms (using pillows) to encourage fluid movement away from arms.

9. *A patient is complaining of intermittent pain in the forearm and upper arm. The I.V. site in the wrist shows no signs of complications and a good blood return is easily obtained. The I.V. solution is running well at a very rapid rate. What is wrong?*

ANSWER: Usually, complaints of pain distant from the I.V. site indicate venospasm. The rate should be *momentarily* decreased and warmth applied to the area of pain. This may stop the spasm, but recurrence is possible. If the patient is willing, try to increase the rate to the ordered flow rate and continue warming the vein. If spasm recurs, the I.V. line should be discontinued and restarted in a larger vein. A larger gauge catheter also may help.

10. *Upon routine observation of a patient's I.V. site, the nurse notices that the vein is cordlike. The I.V. runs well, the site is pink, and the patient states, "It's tender to touch." What is wrong?*

ANSWER: Phlebitis. The I.V. line should be discontinued and restarted in the other arm. A warm compress is recommended to soothe the arm.

11. *A patient with a triple-lumen catheter has an I.V. line running through one port. The other two ports are not being used. Do they need to be heparinized to prevent clotting?*

ANSWER: Yes! The triple-lumen catheter is like three catheters combined into one. Each port must be treated like a separate line. When not in use, each port must be heparinized.

12. *When assisting the physician with central venous catheter insertion, which important points should you keep in mind to ensure optimal use and benefits from the I.V. line?*

ANSWER: Always maintain asepsis when inserting and caring for a central venous line. Be sure the cannula is secured and dressed in natural position. Do not allow the cannula to kink or bend. Also, consider the patient's comfort and activity level. Keep the cannula in a secure position that allows the patient to move as freely as possible. Pulling on the insertion site may lead to mechanical or bacterial phlebitis, so secure the catheter to ensure that the weight of it does not pull on the insertion site.

---

13. *An I.V. line is ordered to run at a keep-vein-open rate. What size tubing would be best for this I.V. line?*

ANSWER: The patient will receive the same amount of solution per hour, regardless of the drop factor. However, minidrip tubing is best: The more drops delivered through a slow rate line, the better. The more movement through this line, the less chance of a clotted I.V. line. Also, it will be easier to count the drops with minidrip tubing. Remember the formula: "minidrip < 50 to 75 ml/hour > maxidrip."

---

14. *Even though normal saline solution was pushed through a line of dextrose 5% in water (D_5W) before giving Dilantin via I.V. push, precipitation still occurred in the tubing. Why?*

ANSWER: Dilantin precipitates readily in dextrose. A thorough flushing of the I.V. line is recommended to clear the tubing of dextrose. Do not hold strictly to the use of 5 ml or 10 ml normal saline solution flush before administering a Dilantin push. It may take as much as four times the amount to clear the line of any medication. Also keep in mind the distance between the cannula and the Y-port where the medication will be injected when flushing the line. Every I.V. line is not the same length, so the amount of solution needed to thoroughly flush a line will differ. In addition, it may be a good idea to flush the line with normal saline solution at a point that is farther away from the patient than the site at which Dilantin is being administered. This helps prevent Dilantin reflux into the D_5W solution.

---

15. *Can any type of total parenteral nutrition solution be administered to a patient with peripheral I.V. access?*

ANSWER: No! The solution prepared for use in a central venous line is much more concentrated with glucose than the solution used in a peripheral line. Central formulas infused via a peripheral line will be extremely painful for the patient, and venospasm, tissue damage, and phlebitis probably would result.

16. *You have a physician's order to obtain a blood sample from an Infuse-A-Port. Is there any way to draw the blood with a straight Huber or Infusaid needle without worrying about needle manipulation?*

ANSWER: Allowing a needle to move around in the Infuse-A-Port is not good practice because it can core the septum, causing I.V. fluid and blood leakage. The use of a T-port between the needle and the syringe will help decrease needle manipulation and will provide enough tubing to use a clamp between syringes. Using a T-port is also less awkward because you will aspirate the blood by pulling toward yourself rather than upward. Ideally, using a 90-degree Huber needle with the manufactured extension attached is the best setup for anything infused or withdrawn from an Infuse-A-Port.

17. *Which piece of equipment should always accompany a patient with a Hickman catheter?*

ANSWER: A plastic tubing clamp or a rubber-tipped hemostat. In case of a leak in the catheter, the hemostat can be used to clamp the catheter between the point of leakage and the body, as close to the exit site as possible, to prevent hemorrhage.

18. *A nurse should always use universal precautions when performing procedures that involve possible contact with blood and body secretions. When inserting a peripheral I.V. cannula, what protection is recommended to prevent contact with the patient's blood?*

ANSWER: Wearing gloves is an essential part of performing a venipuncture. Gloves do not replace hand washing, but they provide a barrier between the blood and you. Hand washing must always follow any procedure involving patient contact, regardless of whether gloves are worn or not.

19. *What is considered to be the normal phlebitis rate?*

ANSWER: The Intraveous Nurses Society recommends that a facility's phlebitis rate should not exceed 5%, meaning that the percentage of catheter removals due to phlebitis should be below 5%.

20. *What is the standard infiltration rate?*

ANSWER: No standards have been set for infiltration, but 20% to 25% is common. It is important to take into consideration the age of your patient population. Older populations will have a higher rate because of their fragile veins. It is recommended that data be collected for approximately 6 months to discover what rate is common for a specific unit, then work to decrease that rate.

21. *The physician orders oxacillin 1 g I.V. piggyback every 6 hours. It is to be mixed in 100 ml of D_5W and administered over 1 hour.*
- *What type of tubing (minidrip or maxidrip) would you use to infuse this piggyback medication?*
- *Which tubing drop factor would you choose?*
- *At which flow rate should you set the I.V.?*

ANSWER: A maxidrip tubing should be used to infuse this piggyback accurately. The flow rate will depend on which tubing drop factor you choose. For instance, if you choose a tubing with a drop factor of 10 gtt/ml, then the flow rate should be set at 16 to 17 gtt/minute; if your tubing has a drop factor of 15 gtt/ml, the flow rate would be 25 gtt/minute; and if the tubing has a drop factor of 20 gtt/ml, the flow rate should be 33 to 34 gtt/minute.

---

22. *The physician orders 1,000 ml of dextrose 5% in one-half normal saline with 20 mEq of potassium chloride to run over 8 hours.*
- *What type of tubing (minidrip or maxidrip) would you use?*
- *Which tubing drop factor would you choose?*
- *At which flow rate should the I.V. line run?*

ANSWER: A maxidrip tubing should be used to infuse this I.V. solution accurately. The flow rate will depend on the tubing's drop factor. If you are using a tubing with a drop factor of 10 gtt/ml, the flow rate should be 20 to 21 gtt/minutes; if the drop factor is 15 gtt/ml, the flow rate should be set at 31 to 32 gtt/minute; and if the tubing has a drop factor of 20 gtt/ml, the flow rate would be 41 to 42 gtt/minute.

---

23. *A patient has an I.V. line in place. There is 350 ml left in the I.V. solution bag, and the flow rate is set for 75 ml/hour. How much longer will this I.V. setup run for?*

ANSWER: The I.V. setup will run for 4½ hours more.

---

24. *One hour before a shift change occurs, a patient is receiving an I.V. infusion at a rate of 100 ml/hour and approximately 250 ml remains in the I.V. bag. What is the best way to prevent clotting in the catheter during a shift change?*

ANSWER: Secure the next I.V. bag, and hang it on the I.V. pole next to the bag that contains approximately 250 ml of solution. Then remove the old I.V. bag and start the new bag just before the shift change (and before leaving the unit). Because all I.V. bags are overfilled by 5%, throwing away the last 100 to 150 ml of solution in the old I.V. bag will not have a detrimental effect on the patient. This way, the I.V. solution will not run out before the next nurse makes rounds.

25. *Standard procedures involving the flushing of I.V. lines and I.V. care according to the placement of the cannula are always beneficial. If all central I.V. lines are to be heparinized, should Groshong catheters also be heparinized as they do not require heparinization?*

ANSWER: Although Groshong catheters do not require heparinization to ensure patency, heparinization is not contraindicated in these catheters. It is more reasonable to have nurses heparinize all central lines rather than expect nurses to identify individual catheters by name in order to maintain them.

APPENDIX D:
STANDARDIZATION OF I.V. CARE

With cost containment continuing to play a major role in health care delivery, many institutions are standardizing I.V. therapy care. This helps decrease costs by promoting the use of similar supplies and equipment for different types of I.V. devices.

The following pages provide guidelines for standardized care of I.V. lines. Note that standardized care is distinguished by the location of venous access (peripheral or central) rather than by the specific type or brand of catheter used. Although the suggested steps in this procedure are typical for most institutions, the amount of saline or heparin used to flush the line may vary. The amounts listed here should be sufficient to flush all catheter types and lengths, regardless of how far the catheter tip is from the port.

Note: If you are considering using these guidelines to establish standardization of I.V. therapy care, first check your institution's procedures and protocols for I.V. care, and be sure to incorporate any necessary changes.

Positive pressure pushes

When using the positive pressure method to administer flushes, begin to withdraw the needle while the last ½ ml of solution is being administered. This technique offers two advantages: it prevents blood from being pulled back into the vein when pulling the needle out of the PRN plug, and it allows the nurse to maintain line patency by flushing with saline solution only.

SASH procedure

The SASH procedure should always be used when working with an I.V. line that is plugged with a PRN adapter. It is also used on all the lumens of a multilumen line.

S = **S**aline flush to remove old heparin from the catheter.
A = **A**dministration of medication.
S = **S**aline flush to remove medication from the catheter.
H = **H**eparin administration with positive pressure.

PERIPHERAL VENOUS ACCESS

This includes hand, arm, foot, and scalp vein sites. All latex ports must be swabbed with alcohol before each use. Alcohol alone is not an appropriate site preparation.

Catheter type

A catheter or needle less than 2 inches in length.

Site care
• Keep the site clean, dry, and covered.
• Change the site and dressing every 72 hours.
• Change soiled dressings immediately.

Flush protocol
• Flush the lines at least every shift for inpatients. Document patency.
• Flush the lines once daily for outpatients. Document patency.
• Use the SASH procedure (see above) after each use of each line that does not have a continuous infusion.
  —*For adults:* Use 5 ml of normal saline solution. Heparin is not needed.
  —*For children age 2 or older:* First use 5 ml of normal saline solution; follow with 3 ml 10u heparin.
  —*For children less than 2 years:* First use 5 ml of nonpreservative normal saline solution; follow with 3 ml 10u heparin.
• Use the positive pressure method (see above) with all flushes administered.

Blood withdrawal
To ensure adequate blood samples, do not draw from peripheral I.V. catheters smaller than 20G.
• Withdraw and discard 2 ml of blood.
• Using a different syringe, obtain an adequate amount of blood for the specimen.
• Flush the line with 5 ml of normal saline solution, using the positive pressure method.
• Flush with heparin for a pediatric patient.

CENTRAL VENOUS ACCESS
This includes subclavian, jugular, femoral, and cutdown access sites. All latex ports must be swabbed with alcohol before each use. Alcohol alone is not an appropriate site preparation.

Catheter type
• Broviac
• Groshong
• Hickman
• Lifeport
• Midline
• P.I.C.C. line
• Triple lumen

Site care
• Use sterile technique at all times.
• Use Acetone first to clean and defat the skin.
• Use Betadine as the last step. Allow it to dry completely.
• I.V. 3000 is the dressing of choice. No gauze under the dressing covering the insertion site.

- Change the dressing every 7 days or as needed.
- If you note drainage at any time, culture the site and initiate daily gauze dressings.
- Change PRN adapter plugs at least every 7 days or as needed if leaking develops.
- Use a Huber needle to access a lifeport.
- Use the proximal port of triple lumens to draw blood, the distal port to administer continuous fluids, and the middle port to administer intermittent medication.

Flush protocol
- Use the SASH procedure (see above) after each use of each line that does not have a continuous infusion.
  —For all patients, regardless of age: First use 10 ml of normal saline solution; follow with 5 ml 10u heparin. Treat all lumens as separate I.V. lines.
- Use the positive pressure method (see above) with all flushes administered.
- Document patency of all lines.
- *For inpatients:* Flush the lines at least every shift.
- *For outpatients with ports and external catheters:* If used, flush daily and after medication administration. If unused, flush monthly.
- *For outpatients with PICC/Midlines:* If used, flush daily and after medication administration. If unused, flush daily.

Blood withdrawal
- Use sterile technique at all times.
- Thoroughly prepare the port, using alcohol first and then Betadine.
- Withdraw and discard 3 to 5 ml of blood.
- Using a different syringe, withdraw an adequate amount of blood for the specimen.
- Flush with 10 ml of normal saline solution, using the positive pressure method.
- Flush with 5 ml of 10u heparin, using the positive pressure method.

SELECTED REFERENCES AND RECOMMENDED READING LIST

Fischer, J.E., *Total Parenteral Nutrition,* 2nd ed. Boston: Little, Brown, & Co., 1991.

Johns Hopkins, *The Harriet Lane Handbook,* 13th ed. St. Louis: Mosby, 1993.

Groenwald, S. (ed.). *Cancer Nursing: Principles and Practice,* 2nd ed. Part III treatment modalities. Jones and Bartlett Publishers: Boston, 1993.

Hastings-Tolsma, M., and Yucha, C. "I.V. Infiltration: No Clear Signs, No Clear Treatment?" *RN* (57)12:34-38, December 1994.

Horne, M., and Swearingen, P.L. *Pocket Guide to Fluids, Electrolytes, and Acid-Base Balance,* 2nd ed. St. Louis: Mosby-Year Book, 1993.

I.V. Therapy, Clinical Skillbuilders Series. Springhouse, Pa.: Springhouse Corp., 1991.

LaRocca, J.C., and Otto, S.E. *Pocket Guide to Intravenous Therapy,* 2nd ed., Mosby-Year Book, 1993.

Trissel, L.A. *Handbook on Injectable Drugs,* 8th ed. Bethesda, MD: American Society of Health-System Pharmacists, 1994.

Weinstein, S. *Plumer's Principles and Practice of Intravenous Therapy,* 5th ed. Philadelphia: Lippincott, 1993.

Yasko, J., Ed. *Nursing Management of Symptoms Associated with Chemotherapy,* 3rd ed. Columbus, Ohio: Adria Laboratories, 1993.

Intravenous Nursing Standards of Practice: Supplement to Journal of Intravenous Nursing (revised). Belmont, Mass.: Intravenous Nurses Society, 1990.

Tenenbaum, L. *Cancer Chemotherapy: A Reference Guide,* 2nd ed. Philadelphia: W.B. Saunders Co., 1994.

RECOMMENDED READING LIST

The following articles can be found in *Journal of Intravenous Nursing.*

Pediatrics

BeVier, P. and Rice, C. "Initiating a Pediatric Peripherally Inserted Central Catheter and Midline Catheter Program," July/August 1994, 17(4):201-205.

Home care

Lockman-Samkowiak, J. "Care of Patients with Acquired Immune Deficiency Syndrome in Rural Areas," July/August 1994, 17(4):206-209.

Grace, L.A., Illian, A.F., and Rivers, M.P. "A Clinical Productivity Management System for Home Infusion Therapy," July/August 1993, 16(4):251-260.

Sanville, M.H. "Initiating Parenteral Nutrition Therapy in the Home," May/June 1994, 17(3):119-126.

Rutherford, C. "Taxol Administration," May/June 1994, 17(3):139-143.

Equipment

Noah, V.A., and Godin, M. "A Perspective on Di-2-Ethyl-Hexphthalate in Intravenous Therapy," July/August 1994, 17(4):210-213.

Camp-Sorrell, D. "Implantable Ports: Everything You Always Wanted to Know," September/October 1992, 15(5):262-273.

Electrolytes

Terry, J. "The Major Electrolytes: Sodium, Potassium, and Chloride," September/October 1994, 17(5):240-247.

Quality improvement

Hayden, L.S. "Risk Management Strategies," September/October 1992, 15(5):288-290.

Gaines, B.S. "Quality Improvement Processes Applied to Infusion Nursing Practice," November/December 1993, 16(6):326-332.

Zonderman, A. "Ethical Dilemmas in Intravenous Nursing: A Problem-Solving Model," January/February 1994, 17(1):12-19.

Williams, E.M., Kelman, G.B., and Jacox, M. "A Regional Survey of Intravenous Therapy Practices," July/August 1994, 17(4):195-199.

Dunavin, M.K., Lane C., and Parker, P.E. "Principles of Continous Quality Improvement Applied to Intravenous Therapy," September/October 1994, 17(5):248-255.

Chemotherapy

Heinzman, K. "High-Dose Ifosfamide and Mesna Therapy in the Outpatient Setting," November/December 1992, 15(6):322-326.

Schulmeister, L. "An Overview of Continuous Infusion Chemotherapy," November/December 1992, 15(6):315-321.

Yucha, C.B., Hastings-Tolsma, M., and Szeverenyi, N.M. "Differences Among Intravenous Extravasations Using Four Common Solutions," September/October 1993, 16(5):227-281.

Yucha, C.B., Hastings-Tolsma, M., and Szeverenyi, N.M. "Effect of Elevation on Intravenous Extravasations," September/October 1994, 17(5):231-234.

St. Germain, B., Houlihan, N., and D'Amato, S. "Dimethyl Sulfoxide Therapy in the Treatment of Vesicant Extravasation: Two Case Presentations," September/October 1994, 17(5):261-266.

Blood products

Gerber, L. "Autologous Blood Transfusion: Why and How," March/April 1994, 17(2):65-69.

Baranowski, L. "Current Trends in Blood Component Therapy: The Evolution of a Safer, More Effective Product," May/June 1992, 15(3):136-151.

Heparinization

Fry, B. "Intermittent Heparin Flushing Protocols: A Standardization Issue," May/June 1992, 15(3):160-163.

Peripherally inserted central catheters

Goodwin, M.L., and Carlson, I. "The Peripherally Inserted Central Catheter: A Retrospective Look at Three Years of Insertions," March/April 1993, 16(2):92-103.

James, L., Bledsoe, L., and Hadaway, L.C. "A Retrospective Look at Tip Location and Complications of Peripherally Inserted Central Catheter Lines," March/April 1993, 16(2):104-109.

Central venous catheters

Lawson, M., and Vertenstein, M.J. "Methods for Determining the Internal Volume of Central Venous Catheters," May/June 1993, 16(3):48-55.

Baranowski, L. "Central Venous Access Devices: Current Technologies, Uses, and Management Strategies," May/June 1993, 16(3):167-194.

Infection control

Markey, J. "Latex Allergy: Implications for Healthcare Personnel and Infusion Therapy Patients," January/February 1994, 17(1):35-39.

Ruschman, K.L., and Fulton, J.S. "Effectiveness of Disinfectant Techniques on Intravenous Tubing Latex Injection Ports," September/October 1993, 16(5):304-308.

Complications

Perucca, R., et al. "Treatment of Infusion-Related Phlebitis: Review and Nursing Protocol," September/October 1993, 16(5):282-286.

Pauley, S.Y., Vallande, N.C., Riley, E.N., Jenner, N.M., and Gulbinas, D.G. "Catheter-Related Colonization Associated with Percutaneous Inserted Central Catheters," January/February 1993, 16(1):50-54.

Richardson, D., and Bruso, P. "Vascular Access Devices: Management of Common Complications," January/February 1993, 16(1):44-49.

INDEX

i refers to an illustration; t, to a table.

i refers to an illustration; t, to a table.

i refers to an illustration; t, to a table.

i refers to an illustration; t, to a table.